no nips no tucks ™

PROGRAMME GUIDE

Notice

This book is not intended as a medical journal. The information contained is intended to help you make informed decisions about your health. It is not intended to substitute for medical advice. If you are taking any prescribed medications, or are new to exercise, please inform your GP that you are embarking on this programme.

Copyright © Yinka Thomas 2007
Published by Angel & Just
www.nonipsnotucks.com
Designed by Reece Sutton
Edited by Michèle Clarke
Illustrations (except page 50) by Carrie Williams
Printed in Malta

ISBN 978-0-9536-436-3-9

Author's foreword

Failing to age is not equivalent to immortality. It is the persistence of pristine youthful health and vigour for as long as an individual lives. In fact prolonged youthful looks long into old age is not a 21st century concept, the Good Book states 'Moses was one hundred and twenty years old when he died. His eyes were not dim nor his natural vigour diminished.' (Deuteronomy 34:7).

The advances made in anti-ageing science will lead to increased longevity as previously incurable illnesses and conditions are made curable. It is establishing a new paradigm in health care, which involves a future where more people will live into old age, producing huge political and economic implications. Most countries' pension systems exist on the premise that people are going to die at a certain age.

These scientific advances will one day replace cosmetic surgery as the anti-ageing treatment of choice. This could also create a global imbalance between developed and developing worlds, or haves and have-nots in terms of these treatments which can prolong life. It could also emphasise the bias that exists in most societies towards the young and youthful. Wherever this new research leads, it may be the beginning of the end of the process that causes the decrepitude of the mind and body, namely ageing.

Yinka Thomas MSc RNutr

To Mum

Contents

Introduction

Yes, you can get older without ageing!

This Programme is not about vainly denying the inevitable – that we will all grow old and eventually die. That we cannot change. But what we can change is the rate at which we age. This Programme will show you how to slow down, halt and even reverse the ageing process.

First, let's make the very important distinction between ageing and getting older. They are not the same thing. Growing older involves accumulating life experiences, acquiring wisdom, learning from your mistakes (hopefully), and of course, accumulating years. To age on the other hand, is to witness the erosion of one's abilities, appearance and vitality. Your skin wrinkles, your joints get stiffer, you don't have as much energy as before, you accumulate fat, you get aches and pains, your hair goes grey and often thins, you don't feel as strong as you did, your libido declines...the list goes on. Although it was always thought that ageing is natural and inevitable, modern science is showing that it is not. Getting older is natural and inevitable, ageing is not – and this Plan will explain how.

There is a growing body of clinical evidence that sees ageing as displaying all of the characteristics of a disease. It is degenerative, it affects every cell, tissue and organ of the body, and, when left unabated, it ultimately results in death. This book will show you how you can successfully 'treat' ageing. How you can incorporate a lifestyle that will keep the symptoms of ageing at bay, and how you can successfully halt and reverse the symptoms if you are already suffering its effects.

What we think of as inevitable parts of the ageing process such as:
- lost muscle tone
- stiffness of joints and aches and pains
- decreased strength and flexibility
- middle-age spread
- tiredness
- wrinkles and thinning skin
- decreased stamina and cardiovascular fitness

are all a result of being sedentary, having hormonal imbalances and a lack of certain nutrients, and consuming certain foods that should be avoided, rather than just getting older.

This Programme will explain the lifestyle changes that you will need to make so that you will very quickly feel and see the effects of these non-invasive lifestyle changes to combat the detrimental effects of ageing. There is no strict eating plan, no painful exercise, and no major upheaval. It has been designed to fit effortlessly into the busy lifestyles that we all lead. But it does require effort from you. If you follow the Programme, and incorporate it into every day of your life, you will be rewarded with youthful looks, vigour, energy and physical strength.

I have researched the very latest in anti-ageing science, and in this book details are given of the most effective, non-invasive treatments and methods that can keep you young looking, vital and energetic, and take years off your appearance. You just need to make that choice!

Ageing is a choice

Yes, ageing is a choice, and the fact that you're participating in this Programme says that you have decided to halt the inevitable journey to decrepitude, which is the final destination if you do nothing. Instead you are embarking on the journey that leads to getting older but not ageing.

Being youthful is not just about looking young. Your attitude is key – being 'like a child' is vital to retaining youthfulness. The traits of curiosity, creativity, enthusiasm and zest for life, adventure, humour, eagerness to learn new things, willingness to experiment and change, open mindedness, playfulness, and love, are all as important to staying youthful as exercising and eating right.

When you meet a person who is friendly and open and willing to establish new friendships, you are left with the impression that that person has a young attitude. However, encountering the opposite, someone who is crusty, curmudgeonly and has a closed mind and heart, you are left with the impression of an 'old fool', 'old something'. Whatever you call them, they're old!

Passion is vital to being youthful. Passion keeps you alive and keeps that glint in your eye. It gives you purpose and meaning. We need to feel that our lives have meaning and significance. Having youthful energy and positive attitudes gives you the tools you need to face new challenges and achieve greater success as time passes. You will wake up eager to face the challenges of the day that lie ahead. You are literally choosing between life and death. Choose life!

Before we get into the Programme, let's look at the markers of ageing.

The markers of ageing

First of all, I am not claiming to have discovered the proverbial Fountain of Youth. The legendary ancient mariners on that quest failed because they were looking without. I believe that the truth is more Wizard of Oz than Ponce de Leon in that the answer to what you seek lies within. With determination, diligence and discipline you can affect those physical and physiological factors that can be positively changed to enhance health and appearance. These factors I call Age Markers.

Age Markers are simply the biological markers of age, and there are a series of Age Markers that this Programme is designed to focus on. Changes in your lifestyle can improve these markers, and, as a consequence slow, stop and even reverse the ageing process resulting in you feeling and looking younger.

See the box below for the Age Markers tackled in this Plan.

- **Metabolism, muscle mass, physical strength, and percentage body fat**
- **Energy/aerobic capacity**
- **Hormone levels**
- **Blood-sugar levels**
- **Immune function**
- **Skin and hair condition**
- **Stress levels**

There are several markers that are not included in this plan such as bone density and blood pressure. I have included those that, with all things being equal, will be negatively affected if you continue to do the same things that you did when you were younger. For example, if you eat the same things and exercise the same amount when you're 40 as you did when you were 20, you will increase body fat, decrease muscle and lose strength, and your skin will age, etc. because these things happen naturally over time as you get older, unless you take steps to stop them.

What are the benefits of taking part?

If you follow and stick with the Programme:
- your metabolism will increase
- you will develop more muscle leading to a more toned body
- you will be physically stronger
- you will lose excess body fat
- you will have more energy
- your skin will be tauter and less wrinkled because of increased collagen production
- you will be less stressed
- your immune system will improve
- it will be easier to manage your weight
- your hair will grow thicker, and restored to its original colour
- the levels of the hormones directly linked to ageing – HGH and DHEA – will normalise, reinforcing all of the above benefits.

All of the above claims are not anecdotal, but have been proven in scientific study and clinical trials.

How does the the No Nips No Tucks Programme compare with cosmetic surgery in price?

Average UK Cost of a Nip and Tuck	Cost of No Nips No Tucks programme (for 3 months)	
Face lift £5,000	Programme guide	£22
	Changing diet	negligible
Liposuction £3,275	Supplements	£90
	Trampoline	£135
	Pedometer	£20
	Water ioniser	£100
Total: £8,275	Total:	£367
	(and the trampoline and pedometer costing £155 will last you a lifetime)	

No nips and tucks?

So why, you may be asking yourself, should I go along the natural route when, after all, a nip 'n' tuck might roll back the years overnight? Well, there are numerous reasons why.

The main one is the possibility of side effects. These include pain, scarring, swelling, bruising, bleeding, infection, sensory change, asymmetry, or worse. Some patients may not be able to resume their normal activities for weeks or months after their operation. Have you noticed how in TV programmes like 'Ten Years Younger', 'Extreme Makeover' or other programmes where they perform liposuction and tummy tucks, you will see the 'before' pictures of the subject in a bikini, tummy hanging out and saggy skin proudly on display. Then in the after pictures, yes the tummy has been sucked and cut away, but she's in a one-piece and a sarong! You will never see the 'after' pictures of a tummy tuck, even months after surgery. This is because everything looks fine with clothes on, but with the clothes off it's a different story – uneven skin surfaces and vivid scarring is what you're not meant to see. A tummy tuck is a major abdominal operation and you're left with a scar running from hip to hip.

Also, you might spot the 'cosmetically enhanced look' that is a tell-tale sign of having been under the knife. The wide-eyed almost expressionless faces are a dead give-away. And many people have unrealistic expectations of cosmetic surgery. They hope that it will 'make them perfect' and when it doesn't, they are left disappointed and often opt for further procedures to obtain 'perfection'.

When you opt for the short-cut, you will not experience many of the benefits of the natural route, such as a greater feeling of wellbeing from the 'feel-good' hormones released when you exercise, e.g. endorphins, and feeling physically stronger, which can lead to more mental strength.

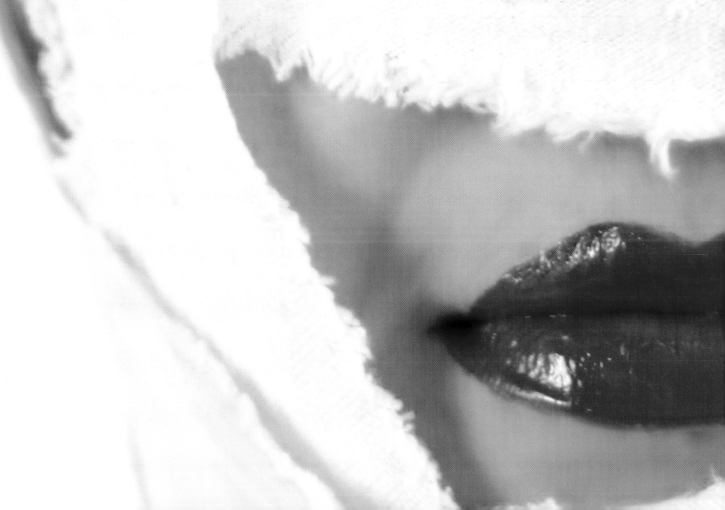

What do I have to do?

The Programme involves four components:
- Dietary modification, but not a 'diet' as such
- A physical activity programme that takes 20–30 minutes a day plus walking
- Taking food supplements, which include a specially formulated anti-ageing blend
- Using the specially formulated skin care products or recommended skincare products.

Monitoring progress

As a means of monitoring your progress on this plan, the measurements you need to take include weight, waist size , body mass index (BMI) and percentage body fat. There is also the option of having your antioxidant levels tested (see the Resources chapter).

You can get your percentage body fat tested at most health clubs and gyms. Mostly they will use a device that you stand on like a bathroom scale; this uses a method called Bioelectrical Impedance Analysis (BIA) to measure body fat. However, using Harpenden Calipers is a more accurate measure – speak to your local health club, or GP.

Try not to weigh yourself while on the Programme (if you can resist). This is not about weight loss – it's about developing muscle to tone the body and increase your metabolism, losing excess fat, improving skin tone and other beneficial changes to make you look and feel younger. Use these indicators as your measure for progress:

- How much stronger and fitter do you feel?
- Does your body look more toned?
- Does your skin feel firmer and is your complexion clearer?
- Has your hair condition improved?

The reason for placing less emphasis on weight is because this Programme is designed to convert fat to muscle, and muscle weighs more than fat. Also,

muscle develops from the inside out so you cannot see the lean tissue that is developing, and you will not see it until you lose the covering of excess subcutaneous fat under your skin when you will then see your improved muscle tone. I say this because you may look in the mirror and see little difference visually. Don't get disheartened. You need to visualise your muscles getting stronger, cells being protected from free-radical damage, and increased collagen production that improves skin tone and hair condition. See in your mind's eye what's going on inside your body.

There is also a 12-week diary at the back of this booklet in which you will find helpful tips and a place where you can tick off daily tasks as you achieve them.

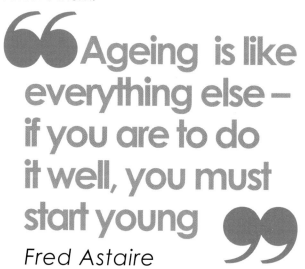

"Ageing is like everything else – if you are to do it well, you must start young"

Fred Astaire

Chapter 1
Why and how we age

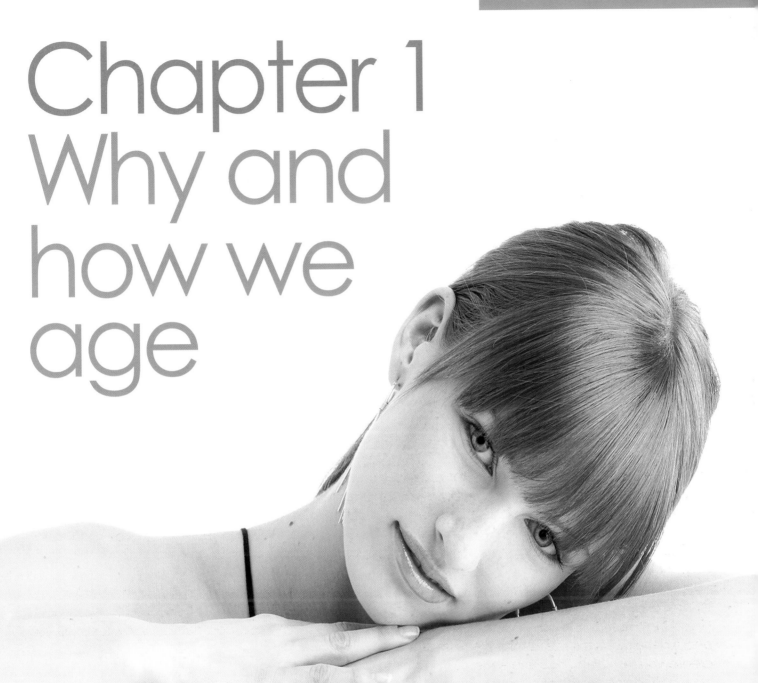

Oxidation
Free radical damage
Inflammation
Hormone imbalance

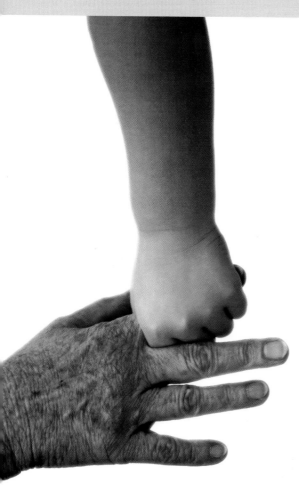

There are various reasons why we age – for the good of the species is one. However, there are possibly hundreds of theories as to how we age, and they all involve the degeneration of certain tissues or processes, such as damage to the heart and arteries leading to heart failure, or free radical damage to cells so that they can no longer function properly.

To think of ageing as inevitable, is like thinking of the body as a machine that will eventually wear out. Living organisms are very different from machines, and this point is best illustrated by the fundamental defining character of a living organism – its ability to heal itself. Flesh heals, skin re-grows, bones repair. A study found that the body totally renews itself every 2 years. The skeleton takes 4–6 months to totally renew, the liver takes 6 weeks, the stomach lining 5 days. Degenerative disease and ageing occurs when cells do not go through normal cell division but mutate, stop dividing or die.

Some cells do continue to divide, but only by turning cancerous. The limited potential for division in a cell is called the Hayflick Limit. However, there exists conflicting evidence to the theory that ageing results from the inability of cells to continue dividing. An example is the decrease in muscle mass that occurs with ageing. This does not result from muscle cells ceasing to divide, but from the death of some cells, and a weakened ability of the remaining cells to increase in size.

The mechanism that controls cell division involves telomeres, which occupy the ends of chromosomes, and an enzyme called telomerase. Telomeres are short sequences of 'junk' DNA, repeated hundreds to thousands of times. Each time a cell divides, all of its chromosomes must replicate so that the two daughter cells have the same genes as the parent cell. Chromosomes become slightly shorter with each cell division owing to the mechanics of DNA replication, and, when a telomere shortens to a critical size, it activates genes that shut down cell division.

Because some cells need to be able to divide indefinitely, such as reproductive cells, they manufacture an enzyme called telomerase, which adds back the shortened ends of telomeres after each cell division, thus allowing limitless multiplication. If there were a way to 'turn off' telomerase, it would arrest the growth of cancers.

Oxidation and the free radical theory of ageing

Free radicals are atoms or groups of atoms with an odd (unpaired) number of electrons, and can be formed when oxygen interacts with certain molecules. This is called oxidation. Once formed, these highly reactive radicals can start a chain reaction, like dominoes being knocked over. Their chief danger comes from the damage they can do when they react with important cellular components such as DNA or the cell membrane. According to the free radical theory of ageing, cells continuously produce free radicals, and constant radical damage eventually kills the cell. When free radicals kill or damage enough cells in an organism, the organism ages.

To prevent free radical damage the body can rely on a defence system involving antioxidants. Antioxidants are molecules that can safely interact with free radicals and terminate the chain reaction before vital molecules are damaged. Although there are several enzyme systems within the body that scavenge free radicals, the principle vitamin antioxidants are vitamin E, vitamin A, beta-carotene and vitamin C. Additionally, alpha-lipoic acid and the trace mineral selenium are powerful antioxidants. The body cannot manufacture these micronutrients so they must be supplied in the diet.

The goal of all research on the free radical theory is to slow ageing by supplying the body with the raw materials that it needs to protect healthy cells, repair damaged cells and regenerate cells to replace dead ones.

Because free radicals do most of their damage when they penetrate the inside of a cell where they can get to the mitochondria – the energy-producing organelles inside the cell, or the nucleus which houses the DNA – it is important to protect the cell membrane with antioxidants. However, because the membrane is composed of fat, in order for an antioxidant to adequately protect the membrane it must be fat soluble. Therefore beta-carotene, vitamin E and most importantly alpha-lipoic acid are important, fat-soluble antioxidants to take regularly.

When free radicals kill or damage enough cells in an organism, the organism ages

Inflammation and ageing

Inflammation is both a cause and an outcome in the process of ageing. It is involved with heart disease, diabetes, Alzheimer's disease, arthritis, kidney disease, stomach and intestinal problems, and other chronic diseases. Inflammation is also involved in disorders of the skin, including cancer. It is a process by which the body's white blood cells and chemicals protect us from infection and foreign substances such as bacteria and viruses.

Injured tissues become inflamed and result in redness, heat, swelling, pain and loss of function. When acute inflammation doesn't shut down, it becomes chronic and causes damage to the injured tissues. Stimuli, such as bacterial infection, trauma, stress-related events, toxic exposures, allergens and chronic viral infections, activate the inflammatory response.

Heart disease and heart attacks are caused by inflammation. It used to be thought that a heart attack resulted from blood vessels becoming clogged with fat and LDL (low density lipoprotein) cholesterol deposited on vessel walls. Now we know that bad cholesterol gets embedded inside artery walls as well, where the immune system sees it as an invader to be attacked. The ongoing inflammation in arteries can eventually damage them and cause plaque to build up causing a blockage.

In some diseases, however, the body's defence system – the immune system – will trigger an inflammatory response when there are no foreign substances to fight off. In these diseases, called autoimmune diseases, the body's normally protective immune system causes damage to its own tissues. The body responds as if normal tissues are infected or somehow abnormal. One example of an auto-immune disease is arthritis.

Hormone imbalance

Hormones are powerful chemical messengers, secreted by special cells in the endocrine organs into the bloodstream where they target particular organs and other tissues of the body. They are made naturally by the body, and keep our bodies working normally. The major hormones implicated in the ageing process are: human growth hormone, dehydroepiandrosterone and insulin.

Human growth hormone (HGH)

Secreted by the pituitary gland, HGH plays a role in determining body composition and muscle and bone strength. It is released through the action of growth hormone-releasing hormone, which is produced in the brain. It works by stimulating the production of insulin-like growth factor, which comes mainly from the liver. Many studies have shown the potential of HGH to strengthen muscle and bones and prevent frailty among older people, and it can be said that HGH holds one of the keys to the ageing process.

A study showed that a group of 12 elderly men managed to reverse their biological age by 10–20 years.[1] They had been given an injection of HGH three times a week for 6 months, and during that period, they reduced their body fat by an average of 15%, while lean muscle mass increased by almost 9%. The participants reported increased energy and libido. However, during the seventh month of injections, several subjects developed debilitating carpal tunnel syndrome, and others developed severe arthritis, high blood pressure, congestive heart disease, and diabetic-like conditions.[2] Although the side effects diminished when the drug was discontinued, so did the benefits. There was also the fear that stimulated cell growth could destabilise the body's mechanisms that regulate cell division, possibly resulting in the growth of tumours. This study led to further research into HGH in an attempt to gain the benefits and avoid the harmful side effects. With these problems in mind, another study investigated the body's mechanisms for producing HGH.[3] It had been thought that the production of HGH in the body naturally decreased as an individual got older; however, the researchers found that the production of the hormone does not decline with age and the body continues to produce HGH well into old age. What actually declines is the body's efficiency in releasing the HGH that it is still producing. They identified secretagogues, which enhance the body's production, release and utilisation of HGH. The researchers found that HGH levels of participants increased by 30% over a period of 12 weeks, and they benefited by other improvements, but without the side effects seen in earlier HGH studies. Secretagogues are available in a supplement called Symbiotropin.

A secretagogue is a compound that stimulates secretion. It is a peptide (amino acid chain) that promotes the release of a target chemical, whether a hormone or an enzyme. Growth hormone secretagogues can cause the pituitary gland to release its sequestered growth hormone, elevating levels to nearer those of when younger. Whereas growth hormone injections cause the body to act as if the pituitary gland has released growth hormone when it hasn't, a growth hormone secretagogue actually causes the release of it.

Secretagogues also come in topical form for the purpose of skin rejuvenation, for example the pentapeptides that we're hearing so much about. When applied to the skin they can stimulate the growth of collagen

How to naturally increase your levels of HGH

- Exercise, particularly exercise that leaves you out of breath, whilst staying well hydrated.
- Get enough sleep.
- Keep blood sugar levels under control.
- Do not eat within 2 hours of bedtime.
- Supplement your diet (see page 97).

Dehydroepiandrosterone (DHEA)

DHEA is produced in the adrenal glands. It is a weak male hormone and a precursor to some other hormones, including testosterone and oestrogen. DHEA is being studied for its possible effects on selected aspects of ageing, including immune system decline, and its potential to help prevent certain chronic diseases like cancer and multiple sclerosis.

DHEA is the most abundant steroid in the human bloodstream. It is often called 'the mother hormone' since it serves as the critical building block from which the body produces other hormones, including testosterone, oestrogen, progesterone, and some 15 other hormones essential for good health, including growth hormone.

Medical research shows that available DHEA dramatically decreases from its peak at age 25–30 until the end of the human life span, where it may be almost non-existent. In fact, no other biochemical in the body declines as greatly. Studies have linked restoring DHEA to the higher levels of youth to increased energy, weight maintenance, increased immunity to cancer, increased immunity to heart disease, improved memory retention, decrease of excess body fat, reduced low density lipoprotein (LDL) cholesterol and enhanced muscle mass, which is so key to any anti-ageing programme.

Studies on DHEA have also shown that it can increase bone density, improve glucose tolerance, enhance feelings of wellbeing, raise HGH levels, improve vaginal tone and moisture, and produce no deleterious side effects in post menopausal women.[4] Another 6-month study with men showed that DHEA significantly increased blood levels of IGF-1 (see box below), produced significant improvements to the immune system, and produced no harmful side effects.[5] A study with patients suffering depression showed that DHEA improved mood, memory and even learning ability.[6]

Insulin-like growth factor 1 (IGF-1) is a crucial blood protein produced in the liver in response to stimulation by growth hormone. IGF-1 provides the best indicator of growth hormone levels and optimal levels are linked to healthy bone, heart, thyroid, skin, and nervous system.

However, not all evidence points to its benefits in anti-ageing. A study published in the *New England Journal of Medicine* in 2006 found that DHEA had no effect on ageing markers such as muscle strength, peak endurance, muscle mass, fat mass and glucose tolerance in elderly men and women. The double blind study involved 87 men and 57 women who were followed for 2 years. Participants showed no change in several markers of ageing – body composition, physical performance, insulin sensitivity or quality of life.[7]

If you still believe DHEA to have an anti-ageing effect, you must be monitored by checking your DHEA levels with your GP both before, and after commencing supplementation. Some people's bodies make large amounts of oestrogen and testosterone from DHEA, while others make smaller amounts, and there is no way to predict who will make more and who will make less. This is a concern because DHEA supplements may cause high levels of oestrogen or testosterone in some people, and with that come side effects such as acne, loss of scalp hair, excess body hair in women, and potentially cancer.

Insulin

Although insulin, when combined in the blood with HGH, is an anabolic (build and repair) hormone and therefore has an anti-ageing function, when it is constantly released as a result of a high refined carbohydrate diet, it is detrimental and pro-ageing. When a diet is eaten that is high in refined carbohydrates, because so much insulin has to be constantly released to get the sugar out of the blood, the body's cells can ultimately become resistant to the hormone, leading to high blood sugar. Uncontrolled diabetes resembles high-speed ageing in that it can lead to atherosclerosis, heart disease, cataracts and blindness, brain degeneration, and stroke. When cells resist insulin, the insulin level outside the cell increases. This increased circulating insulin level has many negative effects, including the following:

● **Inflammation.** Excessive sugar leads to an oxidative process called glycation (see page 31 for more on glycation). Glucose is glycated and becomes a substance called an advanced glycation end-product (AGE) when it is combined with protein and oxygen. Glycation damages the protein and leads to other inflammatory diseases.

● **Hypertension and cardiovascular disease.** Magnesium is an important muscle relaxant and a critical mineral required for over 300 enzymatic reactions in the cell. When the cell is insulin resistant, magnesium cannot be stored. The intracellular magnesium level declines. Without the relaxing effects of magnesium, muscles of the blood vessel contracts, leading to hypertension, Increased insulin in the blood also leads to sodium retention and increase in fluid, worsening the hypertensive state. Without sufficient intracellular magnesium, the energy production cycle in the cellular mitochondria is less efficient and the body becomes more tired and fatigued easily.

● **Angina.** Increased insulin also reduces the production of nitrous oxide. With less nitrous oxide, the vascular system is in a state of vasoconstriction, further worsening the hypertensive stated caused by reduced magnesium and leading to angina.

● **Fat level in blood.** The amount of triglyceride (fat) in the blood is a direct reflection of the amount of sugar intake in the diet. There is almost a direct correlation between triglyceride and insulin levels. Insulin resistance is characterised by high levels of triglyceride, low levels of high density lipoproteins (HDL – 'good') cholesterol, high levels of low density lipoproteins (LDL – 'bad') cholesterol levels.

● **Atherosclerosis.** A blood environment high in sugar is high in free radicals. These free radicals cause the endothelium to be damaged. The damaged endothelium becomes inflamed. This inflammatory process can be measured in the blood and seen by the rise in level of a substance called C reactive protein. As the endothelium's structure is inflamed, it becomes permeable to lipoproteins, particularly LDL and macrophages. These particles will enter into the site of injury, accumulate cholesterol and develop into foam cells. Being adhesive, the cells will attract other unwanted substances , initiating the atherosclerotic process with a fatty streak, eventually leading to plaque formation. The unwanted plaque consists of lipids (fats), complex carbohydrates, blood, blood products, fibrous tissue and calcium deposits, all of which combine to narrow the wall of the artery.

● **Osteoporosis and obesity.** Insulin is a master hormone that controls many anabolic hormones, such as growth hormone, testosterone and progesterone. In insulin resistance, the anabolic process is reduced. Bone and muscle tissue is built upon the command of such hormones, and, when these hormones are reduced, the amount of bone and muscle building is reduced.

● **Reduced sexual function.** Insulin helps control the manufacture of cholesterol that is the precursor of all sex hormones, including oestrogen, progesterone and testosterone, and DHEA. The more insulin resistance, the lower the DHEA level.

Keeping insulin levels low makes cells become stronger, and better able to fight off infection and age-related diseases, such as cancer, dementia and stroke. This can be achieved by balancing your blood sugar levels by managing your diet. We'll look more closely at how you can achieve this in the next section.

Oestrogen

The female hormone oestrogen is used in hormone replacement therapy to relieve discomforts of the menopause. Produced mainly by the ovaries, it slows the bone thinning that accompanies ageing and may help prevent frailty and disability. After the menopause, fat tissue is the major source of a form of oestrogen weaker than that produced by the ovaries.

Testosterone

The male hormone testosterone is produced in the testes and may decline with age, though less frequently or significantly than oestrogen in women. Reduced testosterone levels leads to weakened muscles and frailty.

Melatonin

This hormone from the pineal gland responds to light and seems to regulate various seasonal changes in the body. As it declines during ageing, it may trigger changes throughout the endocrine system.

Chapter 2
The Anti-ageing Eating Plan

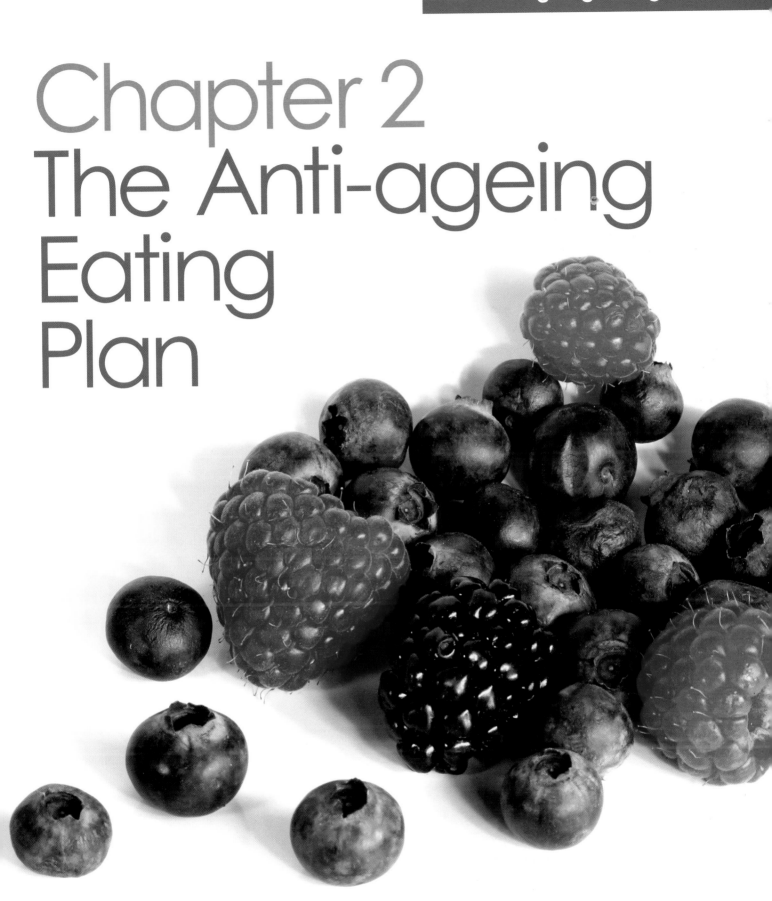

Blood sugar levels
Glycation
Glycaemic load
Glycaemic index
Low-fat diets
Antioxidants

Food can keep you youthful

How we age is largely governed by what we eat, and good nutrition can protect us from the ravages of time and the elements. It can keep our skin supple and toned, and clear from pimples, blemishes and wrinkles. It will provide the antioxidants and other phytochemicals that help to protect the body against free-radical damage, which causes ageing and degeneration. Certain foods can rejuvenate a tired immune system, warding off infection and disease. Other foods can significantly reduce your risk of suffering from cancer, heart disease, diabetes and other lifestyle diseases.

Many of us do not understand the power of food to keep us young-looking. We need to educate ourselves about how what we eat can affect how fast – or how slow – we age, and ultimately the quality and length of our lives. This chapter on food incorporates the latest research on the foods that can keep you youthful and healthy.

There are literally hundreds of diets on the market, the vast majority of them aimed at weight loss. We're told to eat certain foods if we have a certain blood group, to eliminate whole food groups from our diets, to live off cabbage...the list goes on and on. The question is, what do we believe when faced with such a plethora of conflicting theories? The answer is simple – if a diet plan focuses on weight loss as its goal, discard it. If it focuses on maximising your health, or staying healthy, energised and youthful, then read on, because when you're doing the right things to get healthier, losing excess fat will be incidental. The eating plan's goal discussed here is to maximise your health and make you more youthful, and, if you are carrying excess fat, as you follow the Programme you'll find that those excess pounds you are carrying will go as you become fitter and more youthful.

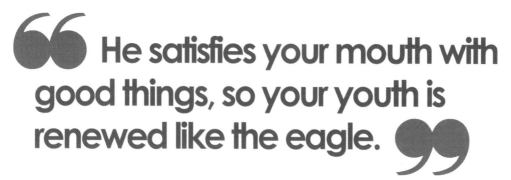 **He satisfies your mouth with good things, so your youth is renewed like the eagle.**

Before we go into explaining how food can affect how we age, look at Table 1, which has a list of the top anti-ageing foods that should feature regularly in your diet. Try to make food from this list the mainstays in your diet.

Food	Properties	Comments
Sardines	An excellent source of omega 3 essential fatty acids, protein and calcium	Salmon also is good for protein and omega 3 fats, but choose red Alaskan salmon or sockeye (tinned is OK) rather than farmed salmon
Greens and other dark green leafy vegetables such as cabbage, kale, broccoli, spinach	Greens contain numerous protective antioxidants and phytochemicals that have anti-ageing benefits including lutein, which has been shown in studies to boost skin hydration and elasticity – and this helps to fight wrinkles. Research suggests that consuming 10 mg of lutein (4 oz of spinach or 2 oz of kale) daily can help the skin look younger in just a few weeks	Spinach comes with higher levels of iron, folate and other protective phytochemicals
Tomatoes	Tomatoes are a rich source of lycopene, which forms the red pigment producing their colour. Recent studies suggest that lycopene has an anti-ageing effect by protecting skin from harmful UV rays. It also helps preserve mental and physical functioning among the elderly and reduces the risk of some cancers	Watermelon and pink grapefruit also contain some lycopene. See the Recipes section for some tomato recipes
Garlic	Garlic is anti-fungal and anti-bacterial, and has been called nature's antibiotic. It contains a chemical called allyl sulphide which research has shown to help fight cancer cells, especially the cells that attack the digestive system, the breast, and the prostate gland. Garlic also has the ability to make blood thinner and less sticky which means it helps to prevent plaque build-up in the arteries.	Kyolic garlic supplements are effective defences against bacterial infection

Food	Properties	Comments
Goji berries	Goji berries contain 18 amino acids including all 8 essential amino acids, and 21 trace minerals, in particular zinc, iron, copper, calcium and phosphorus. They contain 500 times more vitamin C per ounce than oranges – and vitamin C helps you produce collagen that keeps skin firm	
Acai berries	Rich in potassium, iron, calcium, fibre and high levels of anti oxidant anthocyanins that protect collagen from free-radical damage. The acai also contains beneficial polyunsaturated fats and is low in sugar. Acai berries are hard to find but acai juice is available in supermarkets	
Blueberries	Berries are very rich sources of antioxidants	Also eat black grapes, blackberries, cherries, cranberries, raspberries, organic strawberries
Purple and red grapes	Contain the antioxidant anthocyanins, and the phytochemical resveratrol, which protects the heart and blood vessels by decreasing stickiness of blood platelets. It is also an anti-inflammatory	Drink also purple grape juice, red wine (in moderation)
Meat	Meat is high in protein for building lean tissue, and zinc, which helps develop white blood cells to fight off harmful bacteria and viruses	Include lamb, beef, poultry, fortified cereals, yogurt and oysters. Choose grass-fed (free range) rather than grain-fed (intensive farmed) meat and poultry to reduce levels of pro-inflammatory omega 6 fats

Food	Properties	Comments
Extra virgin olive oil	Contains heart-healthy monoun-saturated fats. Rich in polyphenol antioxidants with the most being found in extra virgin olive oil, which can help combat oxidative stress caused by exposure to UV rays	Ground nut oil is also fairly high in the more stable monounsaturated fats so OK to cook with
Virgin coconut oil	Virgin coconut oil is a very stable fat that does not change in chemical structure when heated for cooking. It also enhances thyroid function, boosting metabolism and increasing energy. It also contains the antimicrobial lauric acid, which enhances the immune system	Choose butter instead of low-fat spread, and never cook with polyunsaturated oils such as sunflower oil, corn oil and vegetable oil as they are highly unstable
Flax seed oil	Flaxseed oil, a source of anti-inflammatory ALA, an omega 3 essential fatty acid. Never heat it but have as a salad dressing, poured into a smoothie, or a spoonful on cooled food	An alternative is hemp seed, and Udo's Choice Oil is a blend of essential omega 3 and omega 6 oils plus nutritious coconut oil
Sweet potatoes	A good source of beta-carotene, which the body quickly turns into vitamin A, important for our skin; has other immune-boosting benefits	Choose also carrots, mango, papaya, apricots, cantaloupe melon, yellow and orange peppers, squash, pumpkin
Eggs	Eggs contain omega 3 and 6 essential fatty acids (about 50 mg and 500 mg respectively). Omega 3-boosted eggs contain more. Also contain antioxidants lutein, selenium and vitamin A, plus folate and iron	Choose free-range eggs which contain higher amounts of omega 3 fats

To stay young looking and youthful you need to eat lots of tomato-based dishes and plenty of greens (not just raw but cooked is fine). See recipe section for ideas

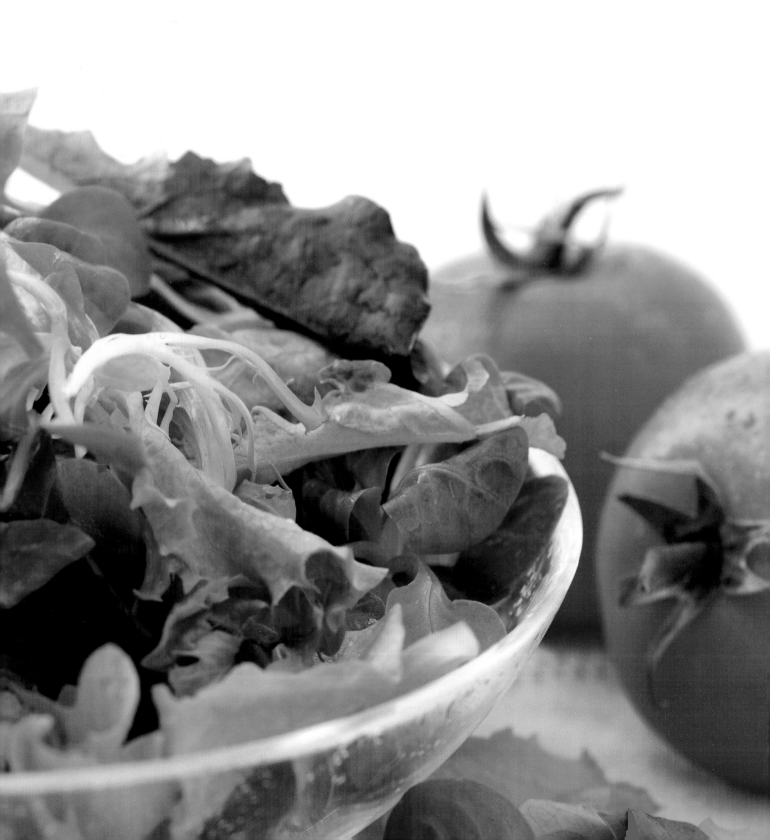

Food	Properties	Comments
Tea	Green tea is high in polyphenols, which protect DNA to prevent ageing. It has potent antioxidant and anti-inflammatory properties	Drink green and black tea. Although it is widely believed that consuming green tea with milk or other dairy products negates its beneficial effects, research has shown that drinking green tea with dairy does not result in a loss of its benefits
Yogurt	Yogurts that contain active cultures are a good source of healthy bacteria for digestive system. Gut bacteria also help make B vitamins, vitamins A and K	Try Kefir, which is a cultured, enzyme-rich food filled with friendly micro-organisms that are good for the digestive system. It is more nutritious and therapeutic than yogurt, and supplies protein, essential minerals, and B vitamins
Turmeric and yellow mustard	Turmeric contains curcumunoids which are powerful antioxidants. Mustard contains isothiocyanates, which stimulate cancer-protective enzymes	Studies have shown that curcumunoids can protect against rheumatoid arthritis, and skin cancer
Kiwi fruit	Higher in vitamin C than oranges	Kiwi fruit is also a good source of the important fat-soluble antioxidant, vitamin E.
Dark chocolate	As well as being a delicious treat, dark chocolate has been shown to have strong antioxidant properties, increase dopamine release and provide flavonoids, which keep arteries healthy	Milk chocolate inhibits the absorption of the antioxidants, and is far higher in sugar so choose the darkest you can and have a square (not a bar) a day to reap the benefits
Xango juice	Made from mangosteen fruit, which delivers a rich source of xanthones, antioxidants associated with ageing	Research has shown that xanthones help maintain intestinal health, protect against free radicals, improve the body's natural defences, and keep joints healthy
Basmati rice	Though not directly linked to ageing, basmati rice is a grain with a lower glycaemic index than white rice so provides a more sustained release of energy and doesn't cause a sudden release of insulin	Also choose other slow-burning grains such as whole grain pasta, brown rice, and many legumes, including chick peas, kidney beans, black beans, lentils and pinto beans have a low glycaemic index

So how can food affect how we age?

Various factors are involved:

● Fluctuating blood sugar levels

● Inadequate protein consumption

● Consuming a very low-fat diet and/or bad fats.

Fluctuating blood sugar levels

The ability of our bodies to control our blood sugar levels declines as we get older. Unfortunately this has two fundamental implications regarding the rate at which we age:

● As our blood sugar levels rise with age, our chances of developing type 2 diabetes increases. And uncontrolled diabetes resembles high-speed ageing in that it can lead to atherosclerosis, heart disease, cataracts and blindness, brain degeneration, and stroke.

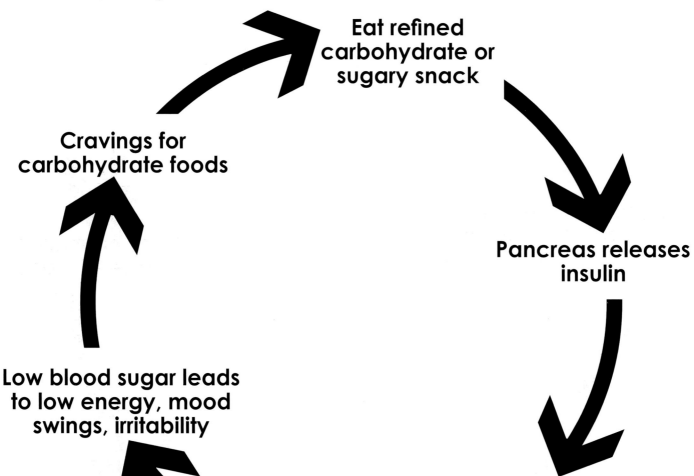

Eat refined carbohydrate or sugary snack

Pancreas releases insulin

Insulin removes sugar from blood after which it is stored in the liver and muscle as glycogen or converted to fat and stored in fat cells

Low blood sugar leads to low energy, mood swings, irritability

Cravings for carbohydrate foods

This cycle can also lead to cells becoming insulin resistant causing high blood sugar, glycation, and type 2 diabetes

● High blood sugar can lead to 'glycation', which occurs when glucose binds to proteins. These glycated products, termed 'advanced glycation end-products' or AGEs for short, literally age you. The affected proteins no longer work properly, degenerate and lead to ageing. Since collagen is a protein, this directly ages the skin.

Science has discovered that age-related glucose intolerance is not entirely due to the pancreas' inability to secrete sufficient insulin, but more to do with a body composition high in fat and low in muscle mass. It also has a lot to do with the types of grains and sugars that you eat. Therefore it follows that you can turn around glucose intolerance and your body's pre-diabetic state, and consequently your propensity to produce AGEs that are instrumental in ageing your body, by *changing your lifestyle*. This state can be turned around by following an anti-ageing eating and exercise plan that will keep you youthful and give you more energy.

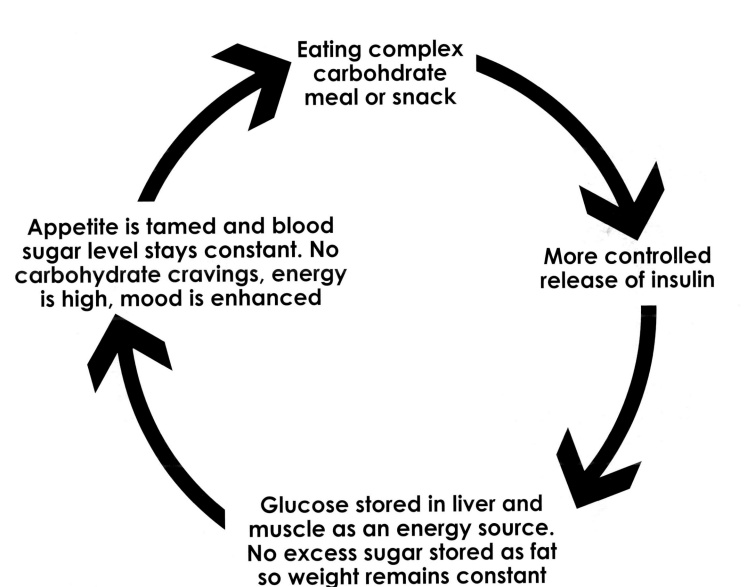

Eating complex carbohdrate meal or snack

More controlled release of insulin

Glucose stored in liver and muscle as an energy source. No excess sugar stored as fat so weight remains constant

Appetite is tamed and blood sugar level stays constant. No carbohydrate cravings, energy is high, mood is enhanced

With this cycle you will age more slowly from reduced glycation

Keeping your blood sugar balanced is one of the most important factors in maintaining energy levels, keeping your weight constant, and staying youthful. No matter how much starch we eat, or don't eat, our bodies try to maintain blood sugar at relatively constant levels.

When our blood sugar is low, you feel hungry and irritable, and the liver will manufacture glucose, which will feed the body, and the brain. When blood glucose is high, for example after a sugary snack, certain cells of the pancreas secrete the hormone insulin. The main target organ for insulin is the liver, which removes glucose from the blood by turning it into glycogen, where it is stored in the muscles and the liver. This may trigger a rapid drop in blood sugar, which makes you feel not only lethargic, but hungry again.

As there is now not enough sugar in the bloodstream, your brain sends a red alert to your adrenals to release adrenalin and cortisol. *Adrenalin* helps release energy from sugar stored in the liver and muscles, and *cortisol* breaks down your own muscle mass to turn it into sugar. Since excess sugar damages brain and body cells, this influx of sugar into the bloodstream triggers further secretions of insulin, which immediately stores away this new sugar into cells.

If you eat lots of refined starches and sugars, there will come a time when there is no more room for glycogen in your liver and muscles. And the high levels of insulin released will turn the excess glucose into fat where it is stored in the fat cells. At the same time the high levels of insulin inhibits the breakdown of fat.

Also, as glycogen stores are constrained by the size of the muscles, this is the primary reason why older people tend to have very low amounts of glycogen in their bodies – they have smaller muscles. Increase the size of your muscles, and you increase your energy stores.

Muscle cells have insulin receptors that are sensitive to insulin. As people get older, they develop too much body fat and lose muscle, and with less muscle there are fewer insulin receptors, and less sensitivity to insulin. So in older people, it takes more and more insulin to have the desired effect of lowering blood glucose levels. And raised blood glucose levels leads to more damage by glycation leading to advanced glycation end-products (AGEs) and further ageing.

Also, if you frequently eat sugars and fast-burning refined starches, the pancreatic cells that release insulin will eventually 'wear out' from overuse, leaving people unable to manufacture insulin any more. This condition is type 2 diabetes, formerly known as 'sugar diabetes. This disease leads to a high blood sugar level and not enough glucose going to other organs. It is dangerous because uncontrolled diabetes is a killer. Coupled with that, eventually the adrenal reserve will also become depleted, and you will suffer from decreased muscle mass, excess weight on the waist, lowered metabolism and premature accelerated ageing.

Inflammation

High blood sugar increases inflammation, which is part of the body's natural response to injury or trauma. Although inflammation is part of the body's natural healing process, too much inflammation can be harmful. High blood sugar makes blood thicker and sticky and it is harder for it to flow freely.

High blood sugar levels also start a chain reaction that produces large amounts of free radicals and 'advanced glycation products' (which we'll look at in more detail in the next section), both of which damage the body. Free radicals stimulate inflammatory responses and people with diabetes develop high levels of inflammation. This strong undercurrent of inflammation increases the risk of other diseases, such as heart disease.

Glycation

Diabetes is such a serious disease because it puts its sufferers in a state of rapid ageing, and this is due to the heightened incidence of glycation taking place in the body. Glycation is the result of high blood sugar levels resulting in a sugar molecule, such as fructose or glucose bonding to a protein or lipid (fat) without the controlling action of an enzyme. Enzyme-controlled addition of sugars to protein or lipid molecules termed glycosylation is less haphazard than glycation. Glycation of these molecules eventually leads to advanced glycation end-products (AGEs).

The higher a person's blood-glucose level, the greater and faster is the damage done by glycation. This is extremely significant in the ageing process because most of the body is made of protein. Protein does more than just make muscle. Enzymes are proteins and glycation can interfere with enzymatic activities in the body; proteins are also instrumental in many other biochemical reactions in the body, play a major role in our immune systems, and direct the process of repair and replication of cells.

Our skin is composed of the protein collagen, which keeps it supple and youthful. When sugars combine with collagen it forms cross-links. These pathological effects are found in the upper and lower layers of the skin. Cross-linked (glycated) proteins are classic characteristics of skin ageing. Cross-linked proteins in the skin results in stiffening, wrinkling and the leathery appearance of older skin.[1]

Serotonin levels

These problems can be exacerbated by the fact that many women suffer cravings for carbohydrate foods around the time of the menstrual cycle. This is largely due to the actions of a neurotransmitter called serotonin. Serotonin is known as the 'feel good' chemical. It is the chemical messenger in the brain that affects emotions, behaviour, mood, thought and appetite, and women naturally have lower levels than men. Carbohydrates can help to raise serotonin levels, hence the craving of refined carbohydrate foods when levels are low around the time of the menstrual cycle. However, these refined carbohydrates have a detrimental effect on our skin, and also promote increased body fat. Another way to increase serotonin levels is to increase consumption of the amino acid tryptophan, which is a chemical precursor

White sugar does you more harm than good

to serotonin. Therefore modifying the diet so that it contains adequate quantities of carbohydrate, protein, fat and tryptophan-rich foods can increase quantities of this important neurotransmitter, and eliminate the cravings that play their part in ageing us. Tryptophan-rich foods include: turkey, chicken, fish, game, cottage cheese, bananas, eggs, nuts, wheat germ, avocados, milk, cheese and legumes (beans, peas, pulses), and there are also smaller amounts in breads, cereals, potatoes and rice. Because tryptophan is such a large molecule, other more easily absorbed amino acids actively compete with it. Therefore in order to divert them and encourage the uptake of tryptophan, it is helpful to moderately raise insulin levels by eating wholegrain carbohydrate foods, such as basmati rice, brown rice, wholemeal bread, and porridge oats, alongside the protein foods.

If brain serotonin levels are low then it can be tempting to reach for foods, and substances, which will give us a quick boost. These include sugary foods, refined carbohydrates such as white bread, bagels and other processed foods, and alcohol. The problem with these foods is that they perpetuate the cycle of cravings so it is important to normalise serotonin levels in order to reduce the need to binge eat and drink.

While serotonin is the messenger, the message needs to be received, and the brain chemical receptors are built principally from essential fatty acids (EFAs), including EPA and DHA. These two are found mainly in oily fish, such as sardines, pilchards, mackerel, salmon, and herrings. Supplements such as omega 3 oil blends and cold-pressed hemp seed oil and fish oil capsules can help supply the body with these essential fats.

In order to keep your blood-glucose level balanced, and to reduce the amount of glycation taking place in the body, you must avoid sugars and refined starches that have a high glycaemic index and glycaemic load.

Glycaemic index

The glycaemic index (GI) of a food is the speed with which the carbohydrate in the food is broken down and turned into sugar to be released into the bloodstream. Sugary foods have a high GI, but not all starches have a low GI. Some starches are fast burning, so will be broken down into sugar quickly. Others take longer to be broken down, giving you more sustained energy and taming your appetite.

The GI also influences how much insulin is released into the bloodstream to stabilise the blood sugar level. For example, if you eat two slices of white bread, which has a high GI, the sugar flow into your system will be rapid. The insulin response will be equally rapid, leaving you feeling lethargic as your blood sugar drops, and again stimulating your appetite.

The GI of a food is also affected by the amount of fat it contains. Fat slows down the conversion of carbohydrate to sugar. Excess insulin also promotes the laying down of fat. You need to keep your blood sugar constant – this will keep your energy level up and prevent fat from being deposited into fat cells.

Try to eat some protein with each carbohydrate to slow down carbohydrate absorption, and prevent rapid rises in blood sugar.

Most foods with a high GI are overprocessed, calorie-dense and short on nutrients. Whole foods usually have a low GI, are rich in nutrients and fibre, and have fewer calories for their weight.

Glycaemic load

Now that you understand GI, there is another term that you need to understand to keep your blood glucose level under control, and that is glycaemic load (GL). This measure was created because the GI has its limitations. For example, let's look at carrots. I have seen articles that tell you to eliminate these very nutritious vegetables from your diet because of their high GI value of 92. However this is misleading. GI is based upon servings containing 50g of carbohydrate, but to get 50g of carbohydrate, you'd have to eat about a 675 g (1½ lb) of carrots. GL takes into consideration a food's GI as well as the amount of carbohydrates per serving. A carrot has only 4 g of carbohydrate; therefore GL is worked out by taking the GI value and multiplying it by the actual number of carbohydrates in a serving.

0.92 x 4 = 3.5

By contrast, a cup of cooked pasta has a GI of 71 and 40 g of carbohydrates giving it a GL of 28.

So GL varies with the serving size.

The glycaemic index of some foods	
Parsnips	97
White rice	87
Potato - baked	85
Cornflakes	84
Cheerios	83
Rice Krispies	82
Morning coffee biscuits	79
Watermelon	72
White bread	70
Wholemeal bread	69
Pineapple	66
Potato - new	62
Ice cream	61
Basmati rice	58
Sourdough bread	57
Oatmeal biscuits	55
Banana	55
Sweet potato	54
Pitta bread	57
Baked beans (tinned)	48
Banana cake	47
Heavy mixed-grain bread	45-30
All-bran	42
Porridge	42
Rye bread	41
Spaghetti	41
Apple	38
Pear	38
Yogurt	33
Lentils	28
Cherries	22
Soya beans	18

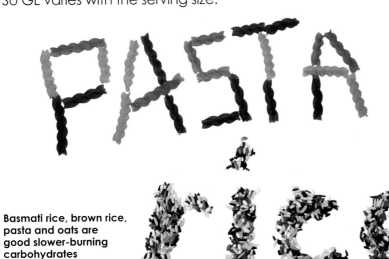

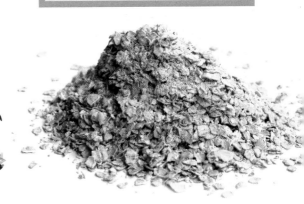

Basmati rice, brown rice, pasta and oats are good slower-burning carbohydrates

Inadequate protein consumption

Protein is used very little for fuel. Carbohydrates and fats are our main sources of fuel for energy. Protein is the body's chief building material. Our muscles, organs, bones, cartilage, skin, hair, nails, blood and antibodies are all made in part from protein, and a good supply of protein is essential for ageing well. Protein is needed in sufficient quantities to enable to body to build and repair tissue, and inadequate protein will lead to accelerated ageing.

Every cell needs protein to maintain its life. The most active protein users of the body are all of the hormones, secreted from the various glands – thyroxin from the thyroid, insulin from the pancreas, and a variety of hormones from the pituitary.

Next to water, protein is the most plentiful substance in your body, and not consuming adequate amounts of protein can lead to loss of skin and muscle tone, stretch marks, sagging breasts, thinning hair, and weak nails. However, this can all be reversed once a plentiful supply of protein is added to the diet.

Protein is composed of 22 amino acids, all vital for healthy tissue. The human body can manufacture only 12 of these 22 amino acids, and 8 are termed essential amino acids and must be derived from food. We cannot build proteins without these essential amino acids. Protein is not one substance, but literally tens of thousands of different substances. The complete proteins that contain the 8 essential amino acids come from meat, poultry, fish, eggs, milk, dairy, cheese and soy. They are, with the exception of soy, anything that comes from animals. Nuts, grains, vegetables and legumes (peas and beans) contain some but not all of the essential amino acids; these are known as incomplete proteins.

How much protein do we need?

Many people consume a very low protein diet, which often leads to tiredness and fatigue. Quality animal protein is important, and by that I mean free-range or organic meat and poultry, because intensively reared animals are fed a diet high in grains that results in increasing the proportion of pro-inflammatory omega 6 fats in their flesh.

Fish is a good source of protein. It contains anti-inflammatory omega 3 fatty acids and is easily digested. However, the problem with fish today is the levels of mercury and dioxins in larger fish.

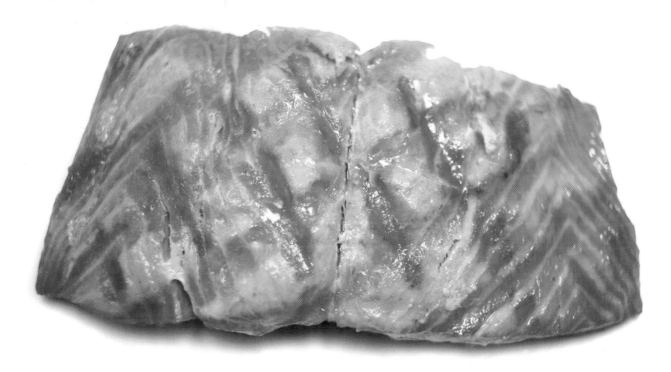

Even government recommendations state that pregnant women should limit their intake of larger fish such as tuna, swordfish and marlin. Therefore I would recommend consuming smaller fish such as sardines and herring, lower down in the food chain and less exposed to harmful toxins.

Table 3 is a guideline for determining your daily protein requirement for ageing well. Pregnant and nursing mothers require up to 40 g more.

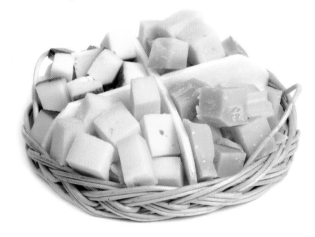

DAILY PROTEIN REQUIREMENTS

Weight (kg)	Protein needed (g/day)
50	50 – 70
60	60 – 80
70	70 – 90
80	80 – 100
90	90 – 110
100	100 – 120

Examples of how much protein different foods yield are
- 3 oz of chicken yields 20 g of protein
- 225 g (8 oz) plain yogurt yields 12 g of protein
- 1 egg yields 6 g of protein
- 250 ml (8 fl oz) glass of low-fat milk yields 8 g protein

It is important to eat regularly and include some form of protein at each meal.

Collagen

Elastic skin is a sign that a person has ample collagen, the strong glue-like material that binds together the cells of your body. Collagen is a structural tissue and it is replaced very slowly. It is made of fibrous protein. In fact, collagen comprises 30% of the total body protein. Its strong white fibres and yellow elastic networks, called elastin, form the connective tissue that holds our body together. Collagen strengthens the skin, blood vessels, bones and teeth. Collagen is one of the most valuable proteins in the human body. A person who has been sick, who has been on an extremely low-protein diet, or hasn't aged well very often sees the muscles in his or her arms and legs begin to sag, which is a sign that they have probably lost collagen.

There is more on collagen in Chapter 4.

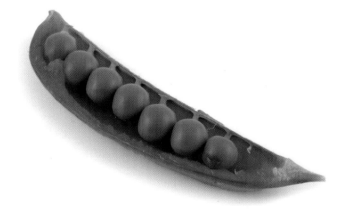

Consuming a very low-fat diet and/or bad fats

When you're trying to lose fat and replace it with muscle, you may think of fat as the enemy, but it's not. We all need fat in our diets, but there are fats that will harm your health, and fats that are an essential part to a healthy diet.

Fat has more than twice as much energy as carbohydrates, yet we are taught to regard carbohydrate as the primary source of energy and told to dramatically restrict fats or cut them out altogether. Yet low-fat diets will not only cause you to age faster, but are bad for your skin. Fat is more than just the best energy provider. It also contains:

● lipids: used in the brain and nervous system, without which we become irritable and aggressive
● sterols: precursors of a number of hormones (including the sex hormones) and the fat-soluble vitamins A, D, E and K. These vitamins can be found in foods, but without the presence of dietary fat, the body cannot metabolise them.

Carbohydrates provide only energy. They have none of the essential components that the body needs to build or repair its tissues. A person fed only carbohydrates would break down muscle and other body proteins in an attempt to keep the essential organs functioning.

There are four kinds of fats:
● saturated (not as bad as you've been led to believe)
● monounsaturated (relatively stable, good to cook with)
● polyunsaturated (highly unstable; omega 3 and omega 6 fats are essential fats, but never cook with them)
● trans (hydrogenated and partially hydrogenated) fats (read all labels and avoid at all costs).

Types of Fats

Saturated fats

Saturated fats such as meat fat, butter, lard, cream, coconut and palm oils are solid at room temperature. They have been much maligned in recent years as being 'artery-clogging' and responsible for heart disease. However, studies show that polyunsaturated are more likely to cause arterial plaque and heart disease than saturated fats. Saturated fats provide a concentrated source of energy in the diet and the building blocks for cell membranes and hormones. Fats as part of a meal slow down absorption giving us a more sustained release of energy. They also help maintain the body's supply of important fat-soluble vitamins A, D, E and K.

Saturated fats are the best fats to cook with because they are highly stable, and their chemical structure does not change when they are heated. This is because all the carbon atom linkages are filled – or saturated – with hydrogen. So they do not normally go rancid. Our bodies make saturated fatty acids from carbohydrates, particularly when we consume a diet high in refined carbohydrates. Blood fat – or triglycerides – do not come directly from dietary fats; they are made in the liver from any excess sugars that have not been used for energy. The source of these excess sugars is any food containing carbohydrates, particularly refined sugar and white flour.

Saturated fats play a vital role in the health of our bones. For calcium to be effectively incorporated into the skeletal structure, at least 50% of the dietary fats should be saturated.[2] This is important for children. They also protect the liver from alcohol and other toxins.[3] Saturated fats also enhance the immune system.[4] Short- and medium-chain saturated fatty acids have important antimicrobial properties, especially lauric acid found in coconut oil, which has antiviral, antibacterial and antifungal properties, and protects against harmful micro-organisms in the digestive tract.

Monounsaturated fats

Monounsaturated fats such as olive oil and peanut oil are liquid at room temperature and become semi-solid if chilled. They have one double bond in the form of two carbon atoms double-bonded to each other and, therefore, lack two hydrogen atoms. Like saturated fats, they are relatively stable. They do not go rancid easily and hence can be used in cooking. The monounsaturated fatty acid most commonly found in our food is oleic acid, the main component of olive oil, as well as the oils from camellia seed, almonds, pecans, cashews, peanuts and avocados. Our bodies can synthesise these fats from other fats. These fats resist damage from free radicals and keep our blood vessels soft and pliable.

Polyunsaturated fats

Polyunsaturated fats such as sunflower oil and most vegetable oils are liquid at room temperature and only become firm if put in a freezer. They have two or more pairs of double bonds and, therefore lack four or more hydrogen atoms. The two polyunsaturated fatty acids found most frequently in our foods are linoleic acid (LA) with two double bonds (also called omega 6) and alpha-linolenic acid (ALA), with three double bonds (also called omega 3). Our bodies cannot make these fatty acids and hence they are called 'essential'. We must obtain our essential fatty acids or EFAs from the foods we eat.

Sources of healthy fats include Wild salmon, walnuts, almonds, pine nuts, flax seeds, olive oil and cod liver oil

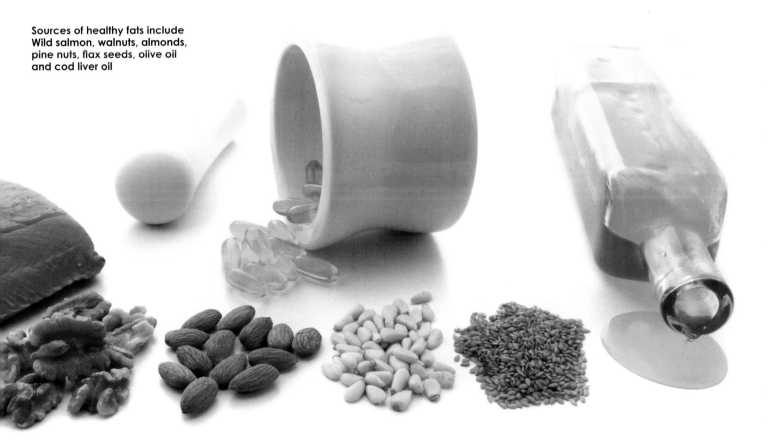

The unpaired electrons at the double bonds makes polyunsaturated fats highly unstable and reactive. They go rancid easily, particularly omega 3 linolenic acid, and must never be heated or used in cooking. Yes, that sunflower oil that we're urged to cook with, because it contains polyunsaturated fats that are good for your heart, actually do more harm than good. Although they are half right in that they are good for your cardiovascular system, this only applies when they are unrefined, cold-pressed and unheated. Exactly the opposite of the processed liquids you find in those clear plastic bottles on our supermarket shelves.

These fats are vital for the brain and nervous system. Omega 3 oils are converted in the body into DHA and EPA – vital for memory, mood, concentration and behaviour. Your brain is 40% polyunsaturated fats, and breast milk is also high at 30%. Omega 3 fats are found in flax and pumpkin seed oils, and in oily fish such as mackerel, salmon, tuna and herring. Omega 6 fats are found in sesame and sunflower seed oils.

Although essential fats are important, our modern diet contains far too many omega 6 fats, which promote inflammation. Excess consumption of omega 6 fats from sunflower, corn and vegetable oils, processed foods and most meat and poultry from animals fed a diet of grains, has been shown to contribute to a large number of disease conditions including increased cancer and heart disease, damage to the liver and reproductive organs, digestive disorders, and weight gain.[5]

One reason the polyunsaturates cause so many health problems is that they tend to become oxidised or rancid when subjected to heat, oxygen and moisture as in cooking and processing. Rancid oils are characterised by free radicals, which attack cell membranes and red blood cells and cause damage to DNA/RNA strands, thus triggering mutations in tissue, blood vessels and skin. Free radical damage also causes wrinkles and premature ageing, and in the blood vessels initiates the build up of plaque.

As the modern diet contains too much of omega 6 fats, it also contains too little omega 3. This fatty acid is necessary for cell oxidation, for metabolising important sulphur-containing amino acids and for maintaining proper balance in prostaglandin production. Deficiencies have been associated with asthma, heart disease and learning difficulties.[6] The best sources of omega 3 are flaxseed oil, hemp seed oil, organic and free-range eggs, and oily fish.

Trans fats

Trans fats or hydrogenated fats are polyunsaturated fats such as soy bean or sunflower oils that are put through a process called hydrogenation or partial hydrogenation that makes them hard. They are used in processed foods as a cheap alternative to butter and to increase shelf-life. Your body treats trans fats as toxic saturated fats – this particular man-made kind does not occur in nature and our bodies have not developed any mechanisms for metabolising or storing them. It simply doesn't have the enzymes to break them down. As a result, once the trans fats from your meal are digested and enter the bloodstream – that is largely where they stay. They circulate in the blood, causing free radical damage and inflaming blood vessel walls. This will ultimately lead to inflammation, atherosclerosis and heart disease. Trans fats may also cause early ageing, skin troubles and other degenerative conditions.

Avoid them – and anything that says 'hydrogenated vegetable oil' or 'partially hydrogenated vegetable oil' on the label. This list includes most margarines, most biscuits, cakes, and chocolate snack bars, junk food and a lot of processed foods.

Avoid low-fat diets

It may go against all you believe and hold true, but a diet including plenty of saturated fat, low in carbohydrates, and adequate amounts of protein with no calorie restrictions, is the best diet that you can follow to maintain weight and muscle mass, and keep you energised and looking youthful. Just look at the evidence, for the past four decades: the general population have been advised to avoid all saturated fats because they 'clog your arteries' causing heart disease and 'make you fat'. However, far from a decline, obesity, heart disease and diabetes have all been steadily rising to the alarming figures that we have today. As the general public have dutifully avoided butter, lard, cream, and coconut oil, choosing instead the polyunsaturated oils and high grain diets, we have got steadily fatter and sicker.

Most modern diets have made people fatter by relying on one overriding philosophy: if you are overweight, you must cut down the calories, starting with the most calorie-dense foods – fat. They therefore work on only one principle: eat a diet of high grain and low fat. And the fats promoted were the processed, polyunsaturated oils such as vegetable, soy bean, sunflower and corn oils, as well as the rise of hydrogenated vegetable oils in processed foods. This way of eating

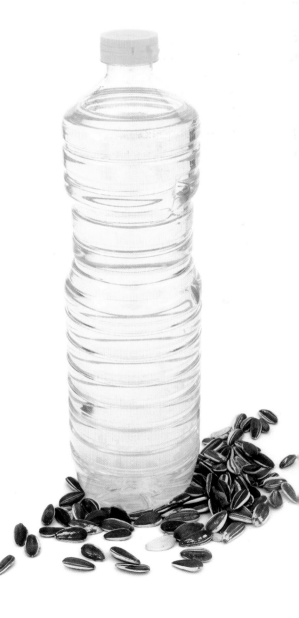

Sunflower oil is an unstable polyunsaturated oil that should never be heated or cooked with. Choose cold-pressed sunflower oils instead and use them in salad dressings or uncooked foods like hummus

has led to western nations' mounting weight gain, and increasing incidence of heart disease and diabetes. There is also evidence that the trans fats in our diets from hydrogenated and partially hydrogenated oils contribute to these diseases as well as cancer.

Fat has a high calorific value, which is why most low-calorie diets restrict fats, but this can be dangerous and self-defeating. Not only does restriction of dietary fat cause the problems already mentioned, it can also cause damage to ovaries in females and infertility in males; kidney damage and weight gain through water retention in the body. When there is little or no fat in the gut, there is nothing to stimulate the production of bile, the gall bladder is not emptied and the bile is held in reserve. This leads to the formation of gallstones. If a fat-free diet is continued for a long time, the gall bladder may atrophy leading to its removal.

A low-fat diet will also age your skin. You will not be getting the fatty acids that help give you beautiful skin, and the fat-soluble vitamins such as vitamin A and D that are important to healthy skin. Also, a diet high in low-fat polyunsaturated products and without a certain amount of saturated fat will lead to 'floppy' cell walls, as the cell wall is mainly composed of fat and polyunsaturated fats are liquid fats. These floppy cells may contribute to wrinkles, whereas consuming saturated fats as part of your diet leads to cell walls with more integrity.

Low-fat diets also lead to faster ageing from free-radical damage to cells, as polyunsaturated fats are the main fats consumed in a low-fat diet and these unstable fats are more likely to turn rancid and produce free radicals. Studies during the 1980s have shown that women who consumed mostly omega 6 vegetable oils had more wrinkles and looked older than women who consumed saturated fat.

Often we're told that for beautiful skin we need to consume litres of water per day. Well that's only half the story. Water does help rid the body of toxins, which can build up and lead to blemished skin. However, the water we drink goes into the bloodstream and out via the kidneys. For water to affect our skin it has to get into the tissues via the cells, and the water in our cells actually comes from metabolising fats. Also, eating adequate amounts of good fats in the diet will mean more fat is available for our oil-producing glands that are the skin's natural moisturisers. So for soft, supple skin you need to drink water, and eat fat.

Acid- and alkaline-forming foods

We often hear about the acid and alkaline forming foods, which means that when the foods we eat are digested, they break down into either an acid or an alkaline end-product in our tissues. This end-product is called the 'ash' and foods that produce an alkaline ash are called 'alkaline-forming' foods whereas those producing acid ash are called 'acid-forming' foods.

The body needs both types of foods. However, alkaline-forming food should predominate over acid-forming ones. Acid-forming foods are meat, sugars, eggs and dairy and most grains, white flour, carbonated beverages, drugs and artificial chemical sweeteners. Over-acidity can force the body to call on its mineral reserves including calcium, sodium, potassium and magnesium, from vital organs and bones to buffer or neutralise the acid and restore balance. Studies have consistently shown that heavy consumers of soft drinks lose the minerals calcium, magnesium, and other trace minerals into their urine. The more mineral loss, the greater the risk for osteoporosis, osteoarthritis, hypothyroidism, coronary artery disease, high blood pressure, and other degenerative diseases.

The availability of convenience and fast foods mean that we eat – and frequently overeat – highly processed, refined foods, as well as those containing artificial preservatives, colourings, flavourings, pesticides, antibiotics and other chemicals.

This type of diet increases toxicity in the body and lines the bowel with a mucoid or slimy substance. This means that waste matter stagnates in the colon where it putrifies, and it can block the passage of other matter, inhibit the full absorption of nutrients, and serve as a breeding ground for parasites and harmful bacteria. It can also produce gaseous compounds, which can make you feel bloated.

Your body works hard to expel these acids in the faeces and urine and through the skin. But when there is acid overload, the body prevents them from circulating in the system and causes damage by extracting minerals and trace minerals from elsewhere in the body. This can produce symptoms, such as lethargy, fatigue, headaches, irritability, weight gain, kidney and gall stones and cellulite, and it can contribute to ageing. So it is essential to ensure a plentiful supply of alkaline-forming vegetables and fruit in the diet.

Get regular

Being regular makes a huge difference in how you feel during the day. It is important that you empty your bowels every day, preferably in the morning. If, during the day, you carry around your waste material, you may absorb some of that waste material into your system. The toxins your body is trying to get rid of will be released back into your system and could weaken your immune system. As that waste matter impacts into the colon, you will be carrying around extra weight in the lower abdomen, and you may feel fatigued, drowsy and irritable during the day.

Do not use laxatives if you are not regular or constipated; instead, to help elimination, ensure you have adequate friendly bacteria in the gastrointestinal tract. Chemicals and pesticides in food and antibiotics destroy these bacteria, therefore it is important they are restored by diet and, if necessary, supplementation. Drinking water is also important, as is eating a diet high in whole-grains.

I don't recommend colonic irrigation – it is not effective at removing the compacted faecal matter in the colon. There are claims that oxygen supplementation can cleanse the colon and remove that compacted faecal matter. These supplements work by introducing 'nascent' oxygen into the intestinal tract, and are meant to remove hardened deposits built up for years on the colon wall. There are no clinical trials that support these claims that I've come across, but plenty of anecdotal evidence that these supplements are effective colon cleansers.

When to go organic

When are we safe to go conventional and when should we go organic? The answer depends upon what crops are the most heavily sprayed with pesticides. The most sprayed crop in the world is not something we eat but something we wear and use on our skin. Cotton accounts for 25% of worldwide insecticide use, making it the most toxic crop on earth. Farmers also use strong synthetic fertilisers because nutrient-hungry cotton plants deplete soils rapidly. That is why I always use organic cottonwool and recommend organic cotton clothing for babies. Regarding fruit and vegetables, surprisingly peaches top that list, although everyone should buy organic strawberries because of the known carcinogen methyl bromide, which is used on conventional strawberries.

This list in the box contains the top 15 of the fruit and vegetables with the most pesticides taken from the ranking developed by the US-based Environmental Working Group (EWG) in 2006.

1. Peaches
2. Apples
3. Sweet peppers (all colours)
4. Celery
5. Nectarines
6. Strawberries
7. Cherries
8. Pears
9. Grapes
10. Spinach
11. Lettuce
12. Potatoes
13. Carrots
14. Green beans
15. Hot peppers

When to go organic

Because most of the pesticides used are fat-soluble and accumulate in the fatty tissue of meats, when you are choosing minced meat products, go organic. Also for similar reasons, the fat in dairy products poses a high risk for contamination by pesticides as animals concentrate pesticides and chemicals in their milk and meat, so go organic for milk, cream and cheese.

Most coffee is grown is countries where there are little to no standards to regulate the use of chemicals and pesticides on food, therefore organic is also a healthier option.

When to go conventional

The next box lists the least pesticide load, so it is safe to buy conventional here.

You can of course peel your fruit and veg; however, valuable nutrients often go down the drain with the peel. The best option is to eat a varied diet, wash all the produce, and choose organic when eating foods from the first list. You could also use Veggi-Wash, a coconut-based product that removes the pesticide residues from fruit and veg (available from health food stores).

Table 4 shows the dietary guidelines to follow, which will determine whether you age fast or slowly.

1. Onions
2. Avocados
3. Sweet corn (frozen)
4. Pineapples
5. Mangoes
6. Asparagus
7. Peas (frozen)
8. Kiwi fruit
9. Bananas
10. Cabbage
11. Broccoli

Table 4 Dietary guidelines – anti-ageing vs pro-ageing diet

Anti-ageing diet	Pro-ageing diet
Eat plenty of fresh fruit and vegetables daily	Rarely eat fruit and vegetables
Eat whole grain carbohydrates such as brown rice, wholewheat cereals, multi-grain bread	Eat refined carbohydrates such as white bread, white flour products, sugar, refined white rice. As well as having a high glycaemic index, these are less nutritious than the whole grain types and will cause inflammation in the skin, which can lead to ageing. Processing adds chemicals and refining takes away vitamins and minerals
Almost never take refined sugar. Sweeten with quality honeys and syrups such as brown rice syrup instead	Eat refined sugar. As well as leading to inflammation and glycation, refined sugar is extremely acid forming, and causes fermentation of the stomach contents, which results in a toxic mass that passes very slowly through the gut. Refined sugar also leaches the body's stores of calcium and magnesium
Eat free-range meat and poultry	Intensively farmed meat comes from animals that are fed a high-grain diet producing high amounts of pro-inflammatory omega 6 meats, and also a cocktail of hormones, antibiotics and other chemicals
Eat a healthy supply of good fats including coconut oil, extra virgin olive oil, unrefined and cold-pressed omega 3 and omega 6 oils	Eat low-fat or no-fat diets, consuming refined oils such as sunflower and vegetable oils, consuming hydrogenated or partially hydrogenated oils
Eat butter	Eat margarine and hydrogenated or partially hydrogenated fats. Man-made fats contain large amounts of chemicals that the body wasn't designed to process

Anti-ageing diet	Pro-ageing diet
Grill, bake and stir-fry	Eat deep-fried foods. As well as being very high in fat, deep-fried foods are often fried in oils that have been heated to very high temperatures and re-used until they turn rancid. The oils oxidise producing free radicals, which are very ageing
Use natural sweeteners such as honey	Use artificial sweeteners such as aspartame, saccharine or Splenda. Aspartame and the chemical flavour enhancer MSG are harmful chemicals, known as 'excitotoxins' which literally excite the neuroreceptors in the brain until they die.
Use herbs and spices instead of flavour-enhancer monosodium glutamate (E621) found in many ready meals, and buy organic	Eat other chemical additives that add to toxic load of the body
Drink juices, smoothies, grape and pomegranate juice, water, moderate alcohol. A little red wine may have some health benefits	Regularly drink alcohol, which dehydrates the skin and speeds the ageing process – try to only have it in moderation. Beer has no health benefits
Eat sardines, wild Alaskan salmon, pilchards, herring	Eat shellfish (crabs, crayfish, lobsters, prawns, shrimps) and molluscs (clams, oysters, mussels, scallops) – these are all scavengers and bottom feeders where toxic pollutants accumulate. This is why, if shellfish 'turns', it can cause serious illness if consumed

Drink water!

Be careful about drinking water left in a car or vehicle in a plastic bottle. These bottles contain chemicals that are known as xeno-oestrogens because they mimic the female hormone oestrogen. However, unlike oestrogen, these chemicals do not break down but instead take up permanent residence in fatty tissue, including breast tissue. Hormone-mimicking chemicals and pesticides have been found in high concentrations in breast tissue that has turned cancerous.

You probably already know this but we need a plentiful supply of water daily. Depending on your size and level of activity we need anywhere between 5–8 glasses of water a day to help purify our bodies and eliminate toxins.

Research suggests that poor elimination of the organic acid waste products in our bodies can contribute to ageing and age-related diseases. The most common organic waste products are acetic acid, ammonia, carbonic acid, carbon dioxide, cholesterol, fatty acid, lactic acid and uric acid. Stress and the modern diet can elevate these levels and can result in arthritis, gout, rheumatism and other conditions. Drinking alkaline water helps our body dissolve acid wastes and makes it easier for the body to dispose of them safely. Alkaline water is not a medicine to cure any disease; however, if consumed regularly, alkaline water can:

● gradually reduce accumulated acid wastes
● increase energy and decrease recovery time
● lower blood pressure
● support the body as it combats the ageing process.

A water ioniser in the kitchen may be a wise investment. Be careful to use alkaline water only for drinking though, because for washing and cleaning our skin, acidic water can help keep our complexions clear and healthy.

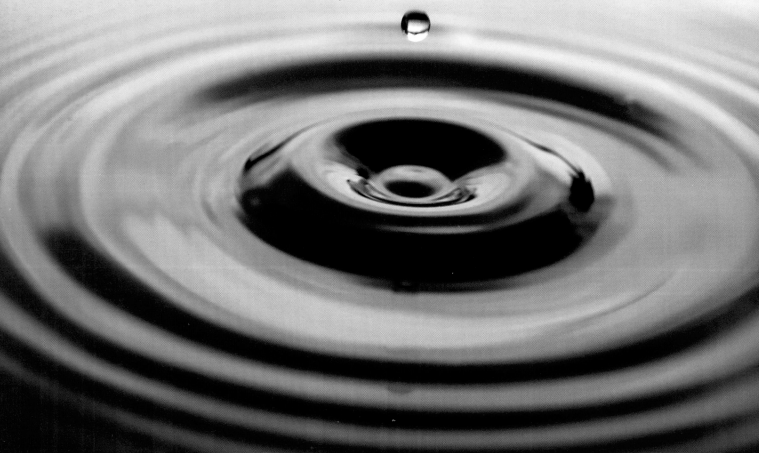

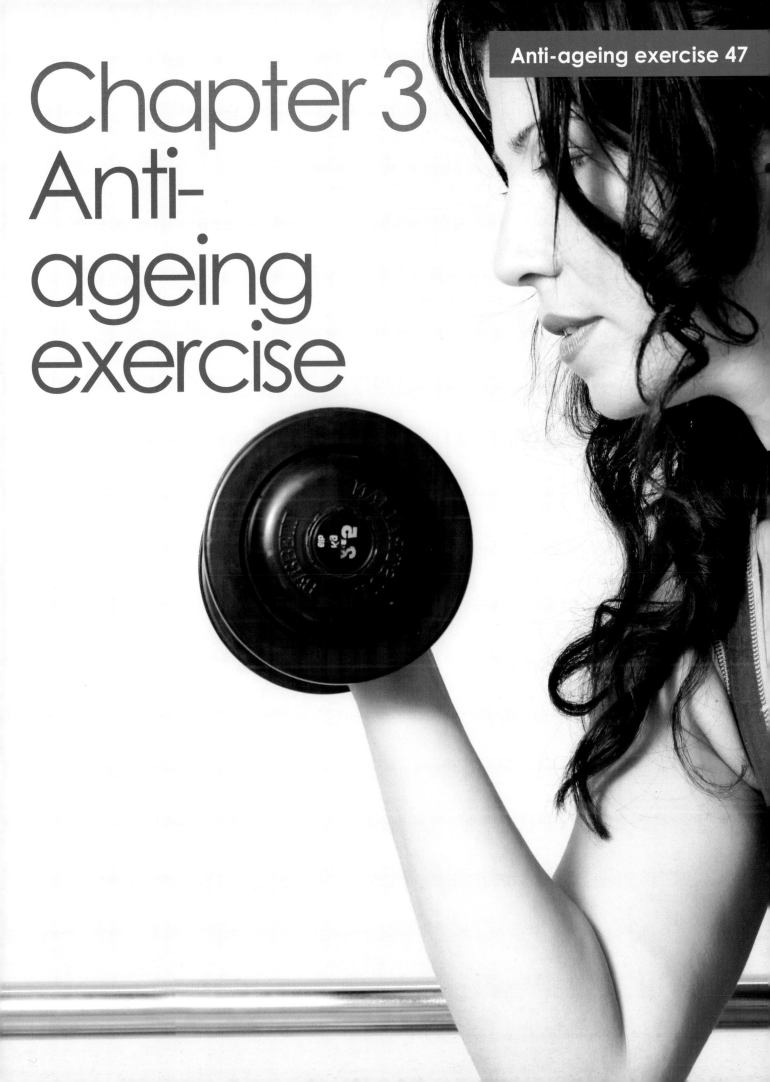

Chapter 3
Anti-ageing exercise

Strength training
Rebound exercise
Stretching
Walking

Let's now look at the exercise plan that will improve the first two Age Markers in the Programme, and have a significant effect on the others. It involves a trampoline (or rebounder), a set of weights (optional), some state-of-the-art walking shoes, and a pedometer.

Exercise can make your face more youthful and halt the move downwards as facial muscles diminish. When fat on the face moves downwards it creates pockets under the eyes, sagging jowls, and a puffy, soft look.

Exercise can reverse all this. The exercise plan used in this Programme is designed to keep you strong and fit. It consists of:

● Rebounding on a trampoline for strengthening and cardiovascular exercise

and

● Toning exercise for strengthening

and

● Walking for cardiovascular exercise.

To get the full benefit of exercise, you need to do both strength training and cardiovascular conditioning (aerobic work). As you get stronger, each pound of muscle you add will burn about 40 calories per day extra of fat. So, if you add muscle, it will help you to lose excess body fat.

The purpose of cardiovascular training is to actually burn calories during the exercise, which is how you achieve the calorific reduction to cause weight loss. And the more of those calories burnt that are excess fat calories, the better the result.

The purpose of strength training is to maintain or increase muscle mass. As stated earlier, the biggest problem with ageing is the loss of muscle tissue, which leads to a decrease in metabolism. With regular strength training, you maintain or build muscle, and this decrease can be avoided.

Why strength training?

The first biomarkers that will change as we get older causing our bodies to age are all interrelated and I group them together as:

- metabolism
- muscle mass
- physical strength, and percentage body fat.

To fully understand their importance in the ageing process they can be dealt with together:

- When you increase metabolism, you burn fat, have more energy, and gain muscle.
- When you have more muscle, you have more physical strength.
- When you are stronger, you have a higher metabolism and burn excess body fat.
- When you don't have excess body fat, you're slimmer and have better body composition and muscle tone, and consequently you look younger.

Metabolism directly controls ageing. Muscle is the body's most efficient calorie burner, and the more muscle we have, the higher our resting metabolic rate – that is, the rate at which our bodies burn calories when we are at rest. Body fat accumulates when we eat more calories than we burn.

As we age, we naturally lose muscle. If we don't challenge our muscles, they will naturally atrophy (waste away) at a rate of about half a pound per year from the age of 20. Even though your weight may stay the same, your body composition will change. You will be the same weight, but have more fat and less muscle. This accounts for the frailty associated with those of advanced years.

A lot of this fat accumulates in the tummy region, and has become known as 'middle age spread'. But a more apt name for it would be 'inactive-muscle induced spread'. Middle age spread, and other signs of ageing are not caused by getting older, rather by not exercising our muscles as we get older.

You can lose weight with aerobics alone, but, very often, you'll end up being a 'smaller' version of a

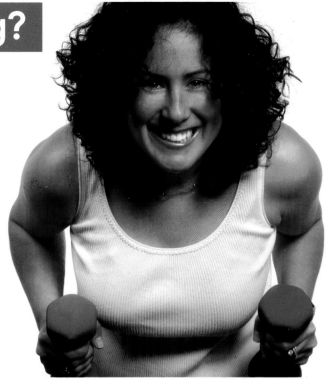

flabby person. Significant muscle tone, definition, and strength are not achievable from cardiovascular work alone. You have to use your weights. You need to train your body to be efficient at calorie burning for the other 23 ½ hours a day when you're not working out. A person with muscle sitting in front of the television is burning more calories at that moment than a flabby person.

Strength training is simply the most efficient way of increasing lean muscle mass. And while time may conspire against you, you can mount a pretty powerful resistance to its ravages with strength training.

Tufts University has been studying the effects of strength training on ageing for many years at their Human Nutrition Research Center on Ageing, and have shown in numerous studies how it can reverse seven major markers of ageing including declining muscle mass, declining strength, increased body fat, reduced aerobic capacity, reduced bone density, poor glucose metabolism, and decreased metabolism.[1]

Muscle is metabolically active, and body fat isn't. All muscles vibrate a little 24 hours a day. When these muscles are 'awoken', they oscillate more, needing to be fed more. This increases your metabolic rate so your body will use food more efficiently.

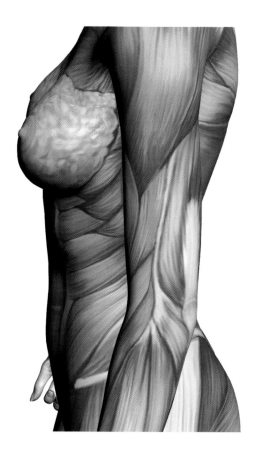

People with a high ratio of muscle to fat on their bodies have a higher metabolism and a higher calorific need. When you have more muscle on your body, even when you're sitting down doing nothing, you'll be burning calories. Fat, or adipose tissue, does not use energy but stores energy; because it doesn't use energy and is metabolically inactive, you'll have a lower metabolism the more adipose tissue you have.

Therefore the more muscle on your body, the less you have to worry about gaining weight. With the fact that muscle is naturally lost as we get older, it follows that unless we strength train, calories don't get burned the way they should, and fat accumulates.

So what is it that determines how much muscle we have?
Two things:
● how much we use our muscles
● the level of muscle-maintaining and muscle-building anabolic hormones in our bodies.

How much we use our muscles directly affects how much muscle we have. The more frequently we use our muscles, the more their tone and size is maintained. 'Use it or lose it' is such a truism (unlike, I'm glad to say, 'no pain, no gain'). And if we push our muscles to their capacity and combine it with other changes outlined in this Programme, the more they will grow and get stronger.

The level of anabolic (build and repair) hormones in our bodies sends signals to our brains instructing our cells, tissues and organs to use the fuel that we consume to build, repair and restore. If, on the other hand, the brain receives 'over-the-hill' signals from a weak, sedentary body, the instructions to the cell tissues and organs are to go into the catabolic state of wear down, break down and degenerate. The primary hormones that put the body into the youthful anabolic state are HGH (human growth hormone) and to some extent DHEA (dehydroepiandrosterone) see page 18.

Other factors that affect strength are that, as we get older, the nerve system that connects our muscles to our central nervous system declines, and the sort of fibres in muscle that are involved in quick actions known as fast-twitch fibres also declines: this, combined with the fact that muscle cells atrophy, results in slower, more measured movements, and a loss in strength.

There are several ways to compensate for a metabolism that gets slower as we get older, thus causing the body to lay down fat. We can cut our weekly food intake by 105 calories every year. In 10 years' time, however, we would have to curb our eating by more than 1000 calories a week. Another option is to add a mile a week – over and above our regular walking workout – every year starting at the age of 30. But by 40, we will have to walk an extra 10 miles per week just to maintain our 21-year-old bodies.

The best option is to add about 60 minutes of strength training per week, plus the other lifestyle modifications outlined in this Programme – and the good thing about this is that you won't have to cumulatively add to your workouts year after year.

A strength training programme will also help to increase cardiovascular fitness. The fact is that, as we age, muscle on our bodies is worth more than money in the bank. Strong musculature keeps you strong, keeps your metabolism high, and keeps you slim and toned, and when you stay strong, you stay slim and look young.

Strong women stay young

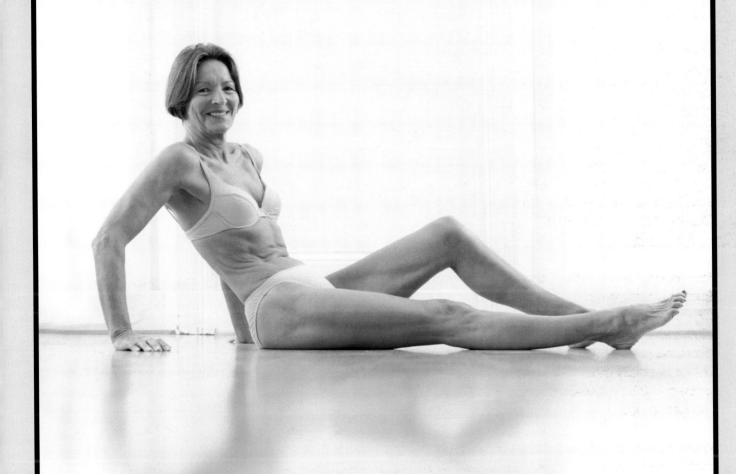

Helen

Helen Hayes has a body that women in their 20s would give their eye teeth for, and legs that go on forever. Yet Helen is a staggering 69 years old. She is a living example of what I've been saying on the last few pages about the importance of muscle on our bodies as we get older, and she illustrates perfectly just how having a strong body keeps you young. Helen, who has just beaten breast cancer has been working out since she was 30, currently trains 4 days per week. in her local gym in East London. Her routine consists of 1 ½ hours of training with weights, and swimming 80 lengths once a week. You don't have to keep to this schedule to look as good as Helen does when you reach her age (or achieve it if you've reached and passed her age already): 30 minutes a day is all it takes, and you can achieve that by rebounding, or as Helen does by lifting weights in the gym (or a combination of both). You will also need to modify your diet as outlined in the previous chapter, and support your body with dietary supplementation.

Why rebounding?

Rebounding, or jumping on a quality mini-trampoline is effective in an anti-ageing plan because of its actions on the lymphatic system and on connective tissue, which help to keep your skin firm and tight. Because of the gravitational effects of rebounding, your body responds by becoming stronger and more efficient. This is one of the reasons why astronauts undergo a trampolining programme before they go into space.

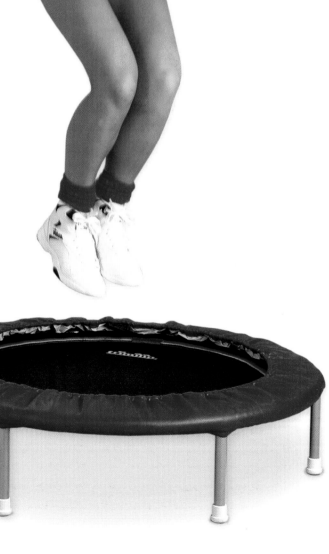

Zero gravity wastes away muscles because there is nothing for them to respond to. Undertaking a form of exercise that increases the gravitational load on the body will strengthen the body. Perhaps the most wonderful thing about rebounding is that it's fun and you don't even feel that you're exercising. Rebounding will very quickly firm and shape your thighs, hamstrings, calves and buttocks. And perhaps best of all, it can give you strong abdominal muscles, this is because you are constantly using your abdominal muscles for balance and stability to keep you on the bouncer.

The gravitational effects of rebounding

Most exercise systems that we are exposed to are designed to oppose gravity. For example, lifting a weight is opposing gravity, Pilates and resistance exercise use bodyweight and gravitational pull; when you walk and run, you first move your centre of gravity in the direction that you want to go, until you start falling in that direction, so then you take another step.

With rebounding, the body experiences complete weightlessness – like an astronaut in space – at the top of the bounce, and at the bottom of the bounce the body experiences the combined effects of gravitational pull, deceleration, and acceleration at the same moment. You will experience a force of 2–3 Gs, which amounts to an increase in your weight at the bottom of the bounce. Every cell in your body will also experience that increase in weight, therefore every cell in your body will respond by getting stronger.

This G loading, is the basic concept of strength training – if you stress a group of cells over and over again (in a muscle), they, and the muscle, will get stronger. So the higher that you bounce (with both feet together), the greater the strengthening effect. It also follows that, if you use the rebounder for jogging or running, the greater the cardiovascular benefits.[2]

G loading stimulates and challenges the entire body cell by cell, and forces each cell to adjust to the increased G force. As a result:

- cell membranes become structurally stronger
- connective tissue strengthens
- bone cells require more bone mineral and the bones become mineralised, denser, and stronger
- one-way valves in the cardiovascular system are stimulated, creating better circulation
- one-way valves in the lymphatic system are stimulated creating better lymphatic circulation (more on the lymphatic system later)
- all anti-gravity muscles – the muscles required for balance – are challenged and strengthened.
- the involuntary muscles of digestion and excretion are stimulated into better performance

Other benefits of rebounding are shown in the box. With rebound exercise, you get fitter and stronger a lot more quickly than with other forms of exercise.

Rebounding increases or improves:

- **Muscle strength**
- **Muscle mass, which makes you more toned**
- **Metabolism**
- **Tendon and ligament strength**
- **Bone density**
- **Balance**
- **Digestion**
- **Mood**
- **Sleep**

Rebounding reduces:

- **Body fat**
- **Risk of diabetes**
- **Risk of osteoporosis**
- **Blood pressure**
- **Cholesterol**

The effect of rebounding on the lymphatic system

When waste material leaves the body cells, it is carried away by the two circulating body fluids: the blood and the lymph. The lymph is formed out of the blood, but contains no red blood cells. The lymphatic system is made up of lymph nodes, tissue fluid, and its associated lymphocytes. It is the fluid that bathes all the body cells, and its primary function is the removal of toxins from the cells, into the bloodstream and out through the kidneys, skin, lungs and colon. It is the body's rubbish collector, the internal vacuum cleaner sucking up metabolic waste, toxins and excess fluid from the extracellular fluid of every organ.

If this flow is impaired, the fluid becomes thick and toxic. The parts of the body that rely on it for elimi-

nation become less efficient and sluggish as they fill with their own waste. This otherwise life-sustaining system now becomes a breeding ground for infection. When the fluid enters the bloodstream, as is part of the normal process, infection can now spread to any organ or part of the body. Many viruses, bacteria and parasites stay locked within the lymphatic system when these conditions are present. The result is cellular degeneration, disease, accelerated ageing, build-up of fatty deposits, and cellulite.

The lymphatic system is not connected up to the heart, so it has to rely upon some other activity to create the necessary pumping action it needs to circulate. The three most important methods of lymphatic circulation

are:
- external massage
- muscle activity
- vigorous exercise.

The lymphatic system is filled with millions of one-way valves, which allow lymph fluid to flow in one way only – usually upward away from gravity. Almost anything that can stimulate the movement of lymph fluid inside the lymph vessels of the system is healthy, but one of the most efficient ways of stimulating the flow of lymph fluid is by rebounding. The up and down rhythmic bouncing causes all of the one-way valves to open and close simultaneously increasing lymph flow as much as 15 times.

There are two ways to cleanse the lymphatic system. The first way is to cleanse the colon, and the second is to practise regular dry skin brushing.

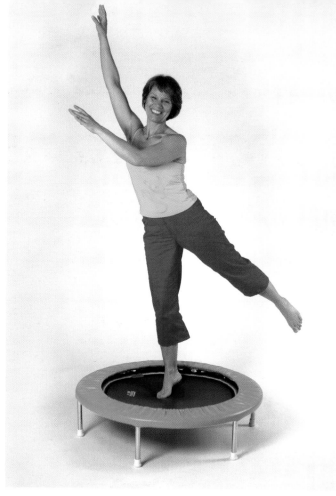

Some basic rules for rebounding include:
- When you are tired, stop. It is important to listen to your body and to do what it tells you.
- Keep your bouncer in sight so that you can jump on it any time for a quick workout.
- Try to do 3–5 minutes (the more the better) of re bounding 15–20 minutes before a meal.
- Use triggers to get onto the bouncer, such as every time you hear a news bulletin, or whenever your favourite soap is on TV.
- Get the rebounding out of the way early. That way, you've got your day off to a healthful start, and you feel good.

- Always start with a warm-up, and end your work outs with the stretches beginning on page 65.
- Take the phone off the hook or turn the ringer off so that you are not disturbed.
- Ensure that you have a clear area in which to put your bouncer, checking for any low hanging ceiling lights.
- Apart from the suggested workouts per week, if you have a spare moment, jump on the bouncer.
- Remember that muscle weighs more than fat so measure your success in inches rather than pounds.

A quality mini trampoline is important

Choosing a good quality rebounder is very important because your whole bodyweight is absorbed into the springs and mat at the bottom of the bounce with every jump you make. Far Eastern-made rebounders that you can buy in most department stores and catalogue stores have low-quality mats that will jar every time you jump, making it an unpleasant experience that you will not enjoy and could cause you pain. These rebounders may be cheap, but they are a false economy because you will end up not using them. You can expect to pay £120 upwards for a quality rebounder. Those in the know consider Trimilin mini-trampolines to be the best on the market. These German-made rebounders use the best quality components and engineering to ensure that your body doesn't jar as you bounce but experiences a smooth bounce – rather like being on a full-size trampoline. See Resources for more on Trimilin Rebounders.

Strong women stay young

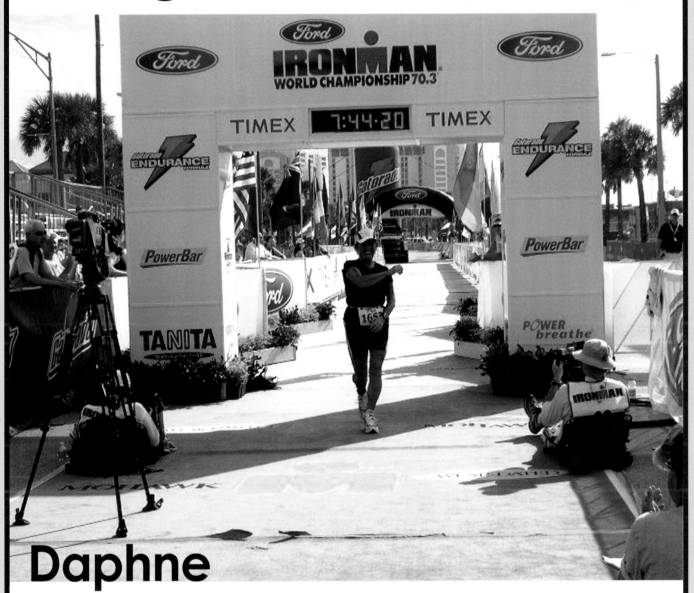

Daphne

Daphne Belt took up the triathlon when she was in her fifties and is now 68. She has been the world champion in her age group five times and has won 28 national titles. She lives in Littlehampton, Sussex, with her husband, Stephen, where they run a triathlon club. She regularly competes in Ironman events, which entail a 4-km swim followed by 180 km on the bike, finishing with a full marathon (26.2 miles or 42 km). It takes her around 16 hours. Daphne trains 4–5 days per week, either on the road or in the pool, except for a 2-week break in the autumn. As a race nears, she'll train for up to 4 hours per session, biking 60 miles and running up to 12 miles. Daphne is truly inspiring, and although you don't have to aim for the Ironman, you can make a huge difference to how you look, and your quality of life as you get stronger and fitter as you follow the Programme.

Using weights

If you prefer, you can combine your trampolining Programme with lifting weights to also reap the benefits of strength training. A humble set of dumbbells is all that you will need to adopt a strength training Programme that will keep you slim, keep you young looking, and keep your muscles and bones strong enough to fend off problems like osteoporosis.

Well-toned muscles give a body shape and form. Muscle toning firms and tightens. It allows you to change your shape, whether you are developing your arms and shoulders to become less pear-shaped or shaping your legs. And being stronger, and having a well-toned, more disciplined body brings positive psychological effects. You will feel better about yourself. Your self-esteem and self-confidence grow. A strong body brings about a strong mind.

You don't need expensive equipment to strength train. You can start off with just a set of dumbbells. The key to buying weights is simple: If you like the way something looks and how it feels in your hands, then buy it. Many manufacturers sell sets of dumbbells with 1 kg, 2 kg and 3 kg weights. This may be a useful purchase if you're a beginner. You can start with the lightest weights, and go up a weight as you get stronger.

The basic exercises

This strength training Programme concentrates on muscle toning. You will learn to isolate each muscle and exercise that muscle until it tightens and strengthens. The strong, shapely bodies that we covet are not attainable without good muscle tone, which you get from strength training.

If you're worried that you'll end up as big and muscular as the female bodybuilders you see in muscle magazines, don't because you won't. Women do not have enough testosterone naturally to achieve those levels of musculature. These women train for about 2–4 hours every day, lifting huge amounts of weights, and taking supplements (drugs and natural) to get to the size that they are. Strength training will give you a firmer, toned, more defined body with a good ratio of muscle to fat.

To get started on a good weight-training Programme that will give you all of the perceived benefits, you need only to do seven basic exercises.

The basic 7 exercises

- Press-ups
- Tummy contractions
- Bicycle manoeuvre
- Shoulder press
- Biceps curl
- Dips
- Lunges

Press-ups

The ultimate upper-body exercise, press-ups strengthen the muscles of the chest, shoulders, arms, upper back and wrist. Strong pectoral (chest) muscles support your breasts and prevent rounding of the shoulders. By working your upper back, you also give your back more width, creating a 'V' shape, which in turn makes your waist look smaller.

Focus on proper technique: Straight back, hold your stomach in, and attempt a continuous movement and full extension of the arms.

Bent-knee press-ups: Keep your back straight and support yourself on your knees and palms. Your arms should be straight and shoulder-width apart. Slowly lower your upper body to the floor, keeping your trunk straight. Rise back to the starting position and repeat.

Standard Press-ups (do these when you are able to easily do 2 sets of 15 bent-knee press-ups): Lie face down on the floor with your palms at shoulder level, fingers pointing forward. Push yourself up until your body weight rests only on your palms and toes. Lower yourself and repeat. To particularly target the chest, place your hands slightly wider than shoulder-width apart; to target the back and triceps, bring your hands close together with thumbs and index fingers touching.

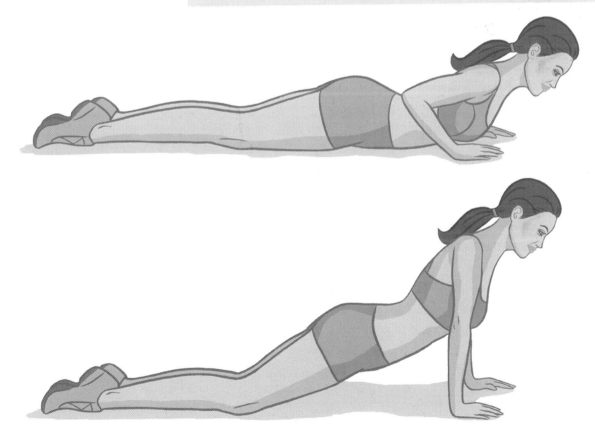

Tummy contractions

The tummy contraction exercises the transversus abdominus muscle, which is one of the most important muscles in the body (excepting the heart of course). This muscle is the body's anchor and is key to holding all other tummy muscles in place. It is important if you want to achieve good posture, prevent back pain, and have a flat stomach. It lies deep inside your abdomen from your oblique muscles at your sides right around your back, and it acts as a corset, helping to prevent wear and tear of the spine, giving us an upright posture, a flatter stomach and a smaller waist. The best method of exercising this hard-to-reach muscle is called a tummy contraction.

On all fours, with hips directly under knees, and hands under shoulders, keeping your back in a natural position and not arched, gently pull your tummy in towards your spine. Hold for a count of 10, increasing to 20, counting out loud to ensure that you are not holding your breath.
Slowly release, taking care not to allow your back to sag.

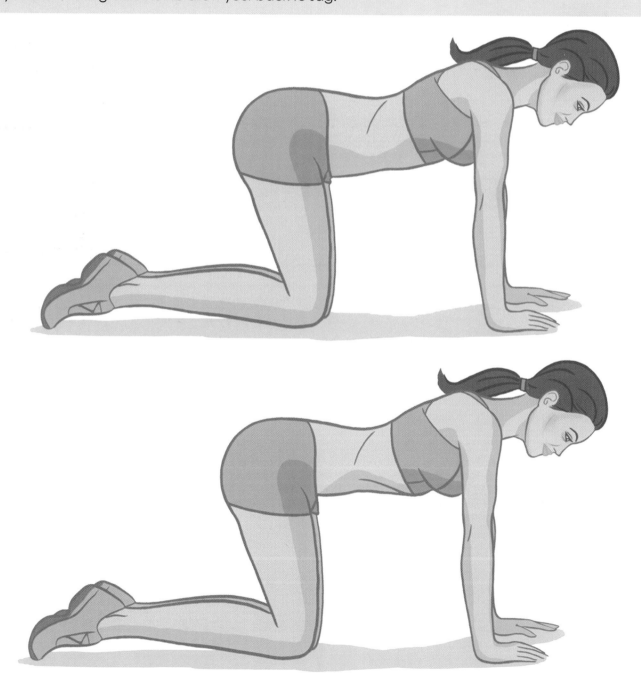

Core strength

The transversus abdominus is the important core muscle that determines the size of your waist. It is your deepest abdominal muscle, and runs from just inside your obliques (at the side of your waist), and right round your back. It connects into the aponeurosis – the connective tissue that covers the front of your abdomen. A strong core means a smaller waist, flatter tummy, better posture and a stronger back. Holding your tummy in is a great way of strengthening your core. I know it's stating the obvious, but it works, and it's surprising how many of us forget to hold our tummies in.

The tummy contraction exercises mentioned are also very effective. Another good way of strengthening the core I've discovered is a home exercise machine called the iJoyRide. It simulates riding a horse and works the core muscles by challenging your balance. See the Resources section for more about the iJoyRide.

Bicycle manoeuvre

Strong abdominal muscles, together with a strong back, complete your torso girdle, and give good posture and a flat stomach. Having a correct posture is one of the best ways to have good health, as you prevent back pain and constricting of internal functions. In a study conducted by the American Council on Exercise, the bicycle manoeuvre was placed second in a study that tested the effectiveness of all known abdominal exercises and popular abdominal exercisers. It was beaten only by the captain's chair, which is a piece of equipment found in gyms.

Lie on your back with hands at your ears, and one leg straight and in the air, and the other leg bent with your knee over your chest. Slowly straighten and bend both legs alternately. Make sure that your abdominal muscles are flat, and that you count out loud to ensure that you are not holding your breath. Start with 20, then continue to increase by 10 as you become stronger.

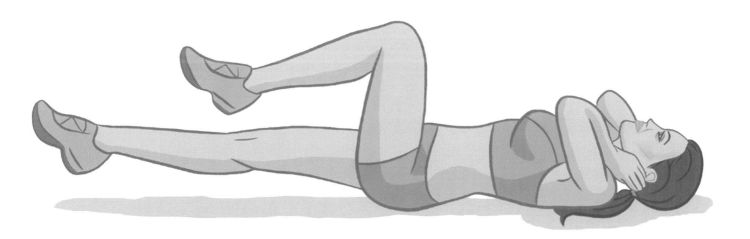

Shoulder press

Also known as the military press, and seated dumb-bell press, it targets the muscles of the shoulders, the deltoids. By working your deltoid muscles, you give your shoulders a square capped off shape, which gives you a more athletic shape, and your clothes will look better on you. Well developed deltoids make you look broader and your waist smaller.

Sit on a chair with your back straight. Holding dumb-bells in both hands, bend your elbows to hold your dumbbells even at shoulder level, with palms facing forward. Press the dumbbells overhead, making sure to keep the weights above your shoulders, elbows slightly bent. Return to starting position and repeat.

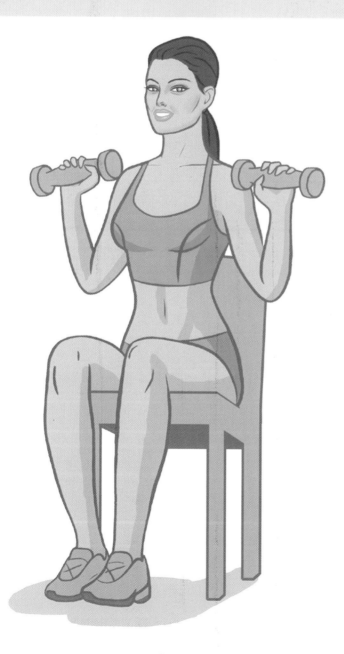
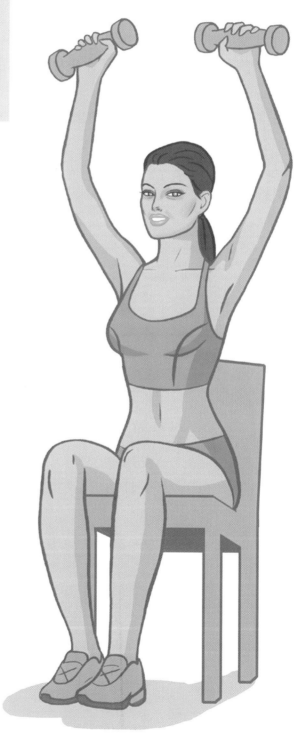

Bicep curls

These target the biceps (front of the upper arms). As well as making you physically strong, good biceps give the arms shape and definition.

Stand with your feet shoulder width apart. With a straight back and head up, hold your dumbbells with your arms resting at your sides. Rotate one arm so that the palm is facing forward, and curl that arm, bringing the forearm towards your biceps with your palm facing up. Then lower the weight, twisting your wrist so that the dumbbell faces your outer thigh, the repeat with other arm.

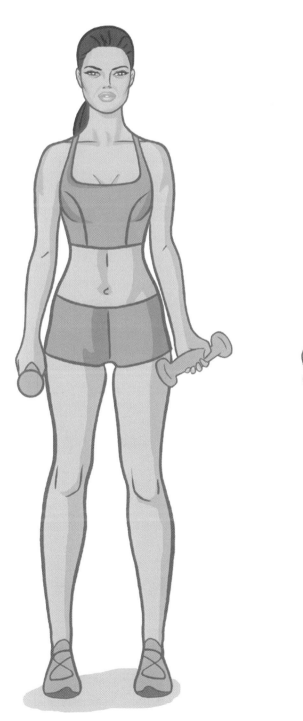
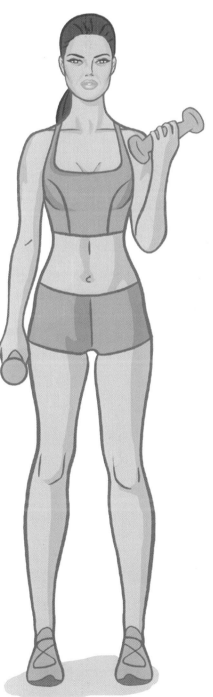

Tricep dips

These target the triceps (backs of the arms). This muscle at the back of your arm, is the one many women feel conscious of – it is the one that flaps when you wave to someone. Strong, firm triceps are a sign of youth.

Sit on the edge of a chair, placing your hands next to your buttocks and fingers facing forwards. Extend your legs so that heels are resting on the floor and legs are straight. Lift yourself up off the chair and slightly forward, then lower yourself towards the floor and lift yourself up straightening your arms. Repeat.

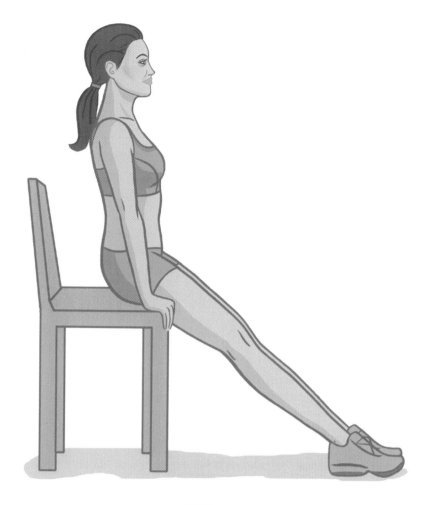

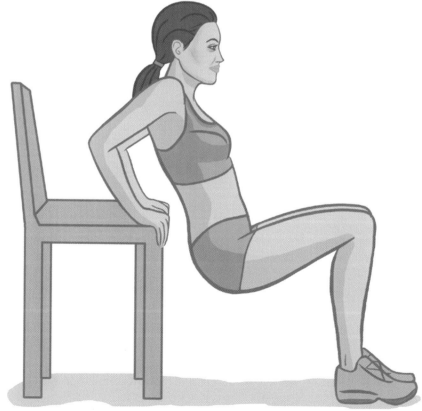

Lunges

Nothing targets the muscles of the back of the leg (hamstrings) and the bottom (gluteus maximus) like a lunge. This excellent exercise also works the abductor muscles (outer thigh), and adductor muscles (inner thigh). There is nothing better than having a tight firm bottom. This exercise is important if you want to avoid your bottom heading southwards as you get older.

Stand straight with your arms on your hips. While keeping your head up and back straight, take a large step forward until your thigh is almost parallel with the floor and lower knee is almost, but not quite, touching the floor. Push yourself back to the starting position then repeat with the other leg. You can do this exercise with your dumbbells for added resistance.

Strength training tips

The general rules for getting started are simple:
- Start with very light weights, weights that let you complete between 12 and 20 repetitions of the movement. If you can't complete 12, the weight is too heavy. If you can easily do 20, the weight is too light.
- Perform between 10 and 15 repetitions (one set) per exercise. Do one set per exercise. Do the routine two to three times a week.
- The basic seven form a great beginner routine. It will teach your muscles what it's like to move against resistance, build neural connections between brain and muscle, and get you on your way.
- Resting time is important. One minute between sets is the optimum since you recover 95% of your strength in that time. Any longer and you will lose the rhythm of your workout, and diminish the benefits.

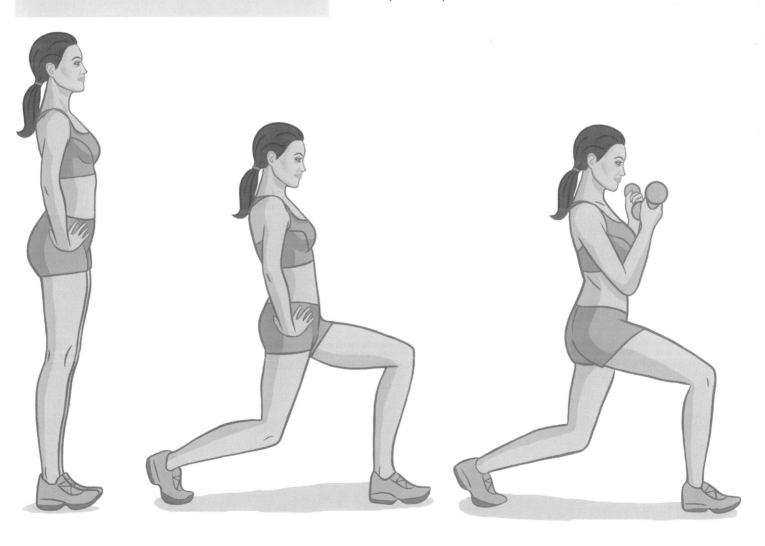

Progressing

For muscles to get stronger, they need to be continually challenged. Once your body makes the necessary adaptations, after about 6–10 weeks of exercise, dramatic muscle change levels off. While you'll still be burning calories, you'll probably stop shedding excess pounds. For continued muscle growth (and to keep burning fat), alternate lighter weight workouts with heavier ones.

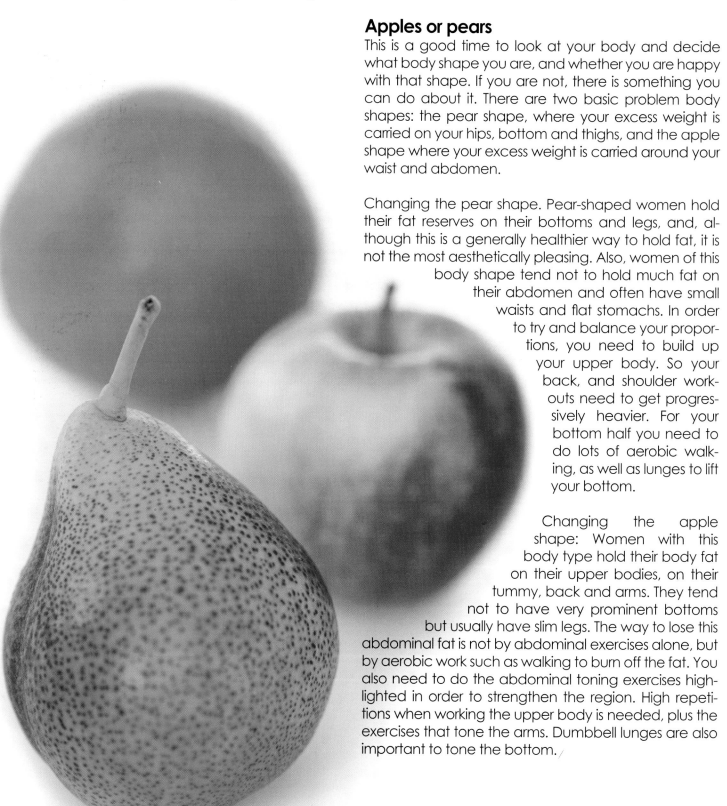

Apples or pears

This is a good time to look at your body and decide what body shape you are, and whether you are happy with that shape. If you are not, there is something you can do about it. There are two basic problem body shapes: the pear shape, where your excess weight is carried on your hips, bottom and thighs, and the apple shape where your excess weight is carried around your waist and abdomen.

Changing the pear shape. Pear-shaped women hold their fat reserves on their bottoms and legs, and, although this is a generally healthier way to hold fat, it is not the most aesthetically pleasing. Also, women of this body shape tend not to hold much fat on their abdomen and often have small waists and flat stomachs. In order to try and balance your proportions, you need to build up your upper body. So your back, and shoulder workouts need to get progressively heavier. For your bottom half you need to do lots of aerobic walking, as well as lunges to lift your bottom.

Changing the apple shape: Women with this body type hold their body fat on their upper bodies, on their tummy, back and arms. They tend not to have very prominent bottoms but usually have slim legs. The way to lose this abdominal fat is not by abdominal exercises alone, but by aerobic work such as walking to burn off the fat. You also need to do the abdominal toning exercises highlighted in order to strengthen the region. High repetitions when working the upper body is needed, plus the exercises that tone the arms. Dumbbell lunges are also important to tone the bottom.

Stretching

Stretching is important before and after strength training, rebounding and walking. A few minutes of stretching will make you less likely to injure your muscles. A tight muscle is a weak muscle, and muscles shorten as they fatigue during exercise. Stretching them afterwards gets them back to the pre-workout lengthened position. Stretching is relaxing and peaceful. It:

● reduces stiffness, muscle tension and soreness
● increases your range of motion
● improves your co-ordination
● improves your posture and balance.

If you don't stretch because you feel tight – you will only get tighter. Here are some stretches to do before and after walking and rebounding.

Pre- and post-exercise stretches

Calf stretch
Stand about 1 metre (3 ft) away from a wall. Place your right foot 60 cm (2 ft) behind your left, and bend your left knee keeping your right leg straight. Keeping both heels on the ground, lean against the wall using your hands to press against it so you feel a stretch in the calf of your right leg. Hold for 25 seconds then repeat with other leg.

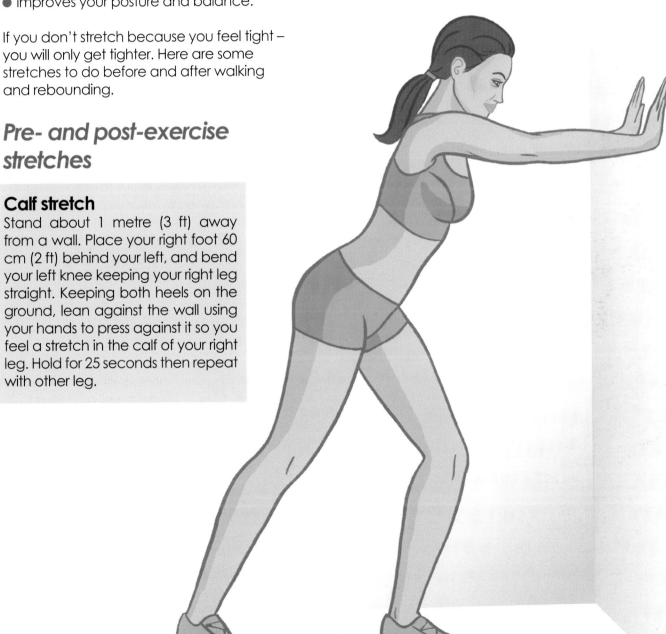

Lower calf stretch

To stretch the lower calf, remain in the same position and bend the right leg, keeping the heel on the ground, so that you feel a stretch in the lower calf. Hold for 25 seconds then repeat with the other leg.

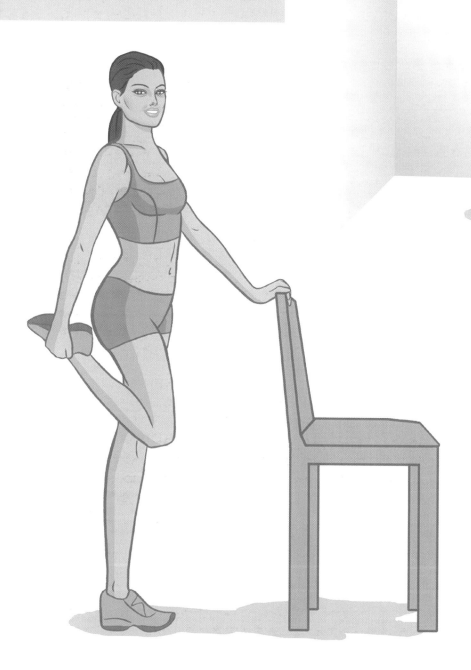

Thigh (quadriceps) stretch

Using the back of a chair or a wall to balance, steady yourself with your left hand, bend your right leg behind you, holding it in your right hand. Pull your foot towards your buttocks and you'll feel a stretch in the front of your right thigh. Hold for 25 seconds or longer then repeat with the other leg.

Hamstring stretch

Place the back of your right leg on your trampoline. Don't lock your standing leg, it should be relaxed and slightly bent. Slowly bend forward towards your right knee, feeling the stretch in your right hamstring. Hold for 25 seconds or longer, and as you become fitter, you can lean more over your knee for a greater stretch. Repeat with other leg.

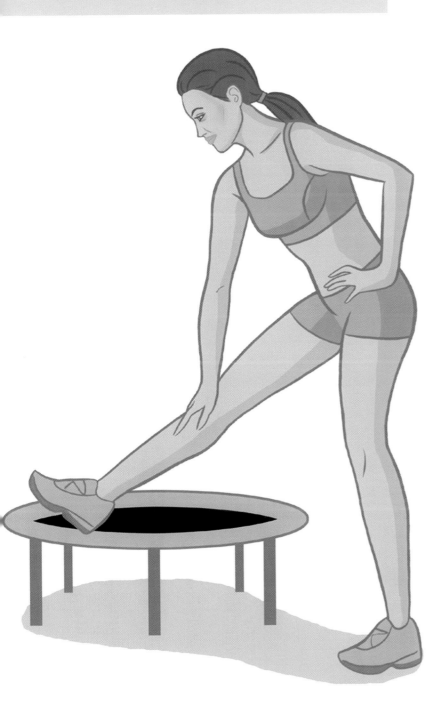

Stretches to do after strength training

Try to do these stretches before and after strength training, holding each stretch for between 10 and 20 seconds.

Start by loosening and relaxing the shoulders by slowly rotating them backwards until you feel looser, then change direction.

Chest stretch

Stand in a doorway with one foot slightly in front of the other. Extend your arms, placing your hands on the doorframe, and lean forward, feeling the stretch in your chest. You can stretch different parts of your chest by placing your arms higher and lower down the wall.

Back stretch

Sit comfortably on a chair and place your hands on the opposite shoulder. With abdominals held in, lean over your knees, relaxing your back muscles and feeling the stretch in the upper back.

Hip flexor stretch

Get down on one knee in the marriage proposal position. Lean forward over your front leg and with your hands at either side for balance, slightly slide your back leg further back and you should feel a stretch in the hip flexor of your back leg. Repeat with other leg.

Also do the thigh stretch, hamstring stretch, and calf stretch.

Buying equipment
See suppliers in resources section.

Aerobic exercise - Walking

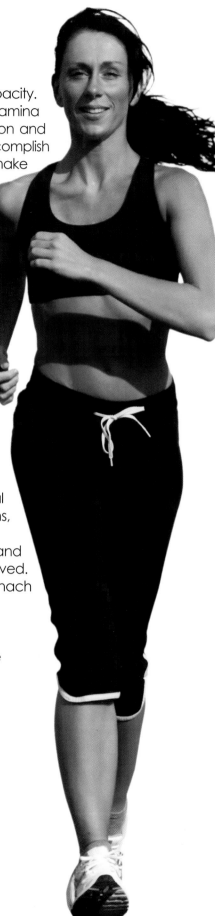

This is important too. There's a difference between energy and aerobic capacity. Energy is the term that we use to describe variations in mental and physical stamina and motivation. The level of it determines our capacity and ability to function and do work, and the amount we have has a direct relation on our ability to accomplish tasks and goals. Physical energy is determined at the cellular level. Our cells make energy through oxidation – the combustion of the fuel we eat and the air we breathe. Your aerobic capacity is your body's ability to process oxygen – that is, breathe it in and deliver it in the blood – via the heart, to all parts of the body. The higher your aerobic capacity, the more energy you can produce and, consequently, the greater your physical stamina. So although energy and aerobic capacity are closely related, they are not the same.

Unfortunately, both energy and aerobic capacity decline with age, and these two occurrences result in the age-related fatigue that many of us feel as we get older. However, the good news now is that science can not only tell us why our energy and aerobic capacity decline as we get older, but also tell us how we can resist the inevitability of tiredness and fatigue by simple lifestyle modifications.

Energy is generated in the cell in microscopic energy 'factories' called mitochondria; however, free radicals can damage the mitochondria, resulting in lower energy produced. A key study, however, showed that it was possible to prevent the damage to mitochondria by ingesting two nutrients – alpha-lipoic acid and acetyl-L-carnitine to boost the activity of a mitochondrial enzyme critical for energy production. Initially tested in rats, then on humans, scientists showed that the boosting of this enzyme reversed the inevitable decline from reduced energy production and led to increased physical and mental energy. Not only did natural vigour return, but memory also improved. These two nutrients are found in foods such as red meat, offal, broccoli, spinach and milk, and there is more about their benefits in the Supplements section.

Aerobic capacity doesn't have to decline with age. It can be improved by regular aerobic exercise. Exercising aerobically when you're older causes the muscle cells – not the cardiovascular system – to consume more oxygen, increasing fitness. And the more muscle you have to demand oxygen, the greater your oxygen metabolism and aerobic capacity.

Aerobic conditioning can:
- help you to burn calories and raise your metabolic rate
- tone the muscles, especially in the abdominal area
- give you a 'high' from the body's 'feel good' hormones (endorphins), which are released when you exercise
- give you an emotional lift
- make your heart and lungs work more efficiently
- help to tame the appetite
- help you relax
- decrease your stress levels
- help you sleep more soundly and deeply.

Why walking?

The best type of aerobic conditioning is that which:

- is most efficient at burning fat
- is as intensive as you want to make it
- is least injurious to joints for even the overweight, and the beginner
- is enjoyable and that which you can perform regularly without fatiguing yourself
- is freely accessible and cost effective
- can include partners, and other family members so can bring a family closer together.

– and that exercise is walking. I strongly advocate the importance of walking. It is low risk – the impact of brisk walking is only about 1.3 times your body weight, compared with high impact jogging and running, which have an impact of approximately 3 times your body weight. It is also one of the best exercises for strengthening bones, controlling weight, toning the leg muscles, maintaining good posture and improving positive self-image. Walking also helps to slow the ageing process.

Walk your way to fitness

Walking is the best way to burn fat. When I first discovered this I thought it couldn't be right. Surely to burn fat efficiently, the exercise has got to hurt? Thankfully, 'no pain no gain' is a myth ('use it or lose it' rings true though). When you feel pain doing high impact exercises, what you are feeling is the effect of lactic acid on the muscles. Lactic acid is a substance produced in the muscles when they become fatigued. You are not burning fat.

To lose weight, it's more important to build up time than speed. Walking at a moderate pace yields longer workouts with less soreness. You cover more distance and burn off more fat.

The pros and cons of high-intensity versus low-intensity workouts are listed in the table.

Pros	Cons
High-intensity workouts burn the most calories per minute – important if you have limited time	You are more likely to cut your workouts or give up completely if you were required to do 3 high intensity workouts per week
Increased workout intensity usually means increased fitness levels	You cannot sustain a longer workout, i.e. moderate walking can be sustained for up to 2 hours or even longer. High intensity workouts can only be sustained for 30–45 minutes if you're already fit. Only serious athletes can go on for longer
	The higher the intensity, the greater the risk of injury

Benefits of low-intensity workouts

- Many people find low intensity more enjoyable and will therefore exercise more consistently.
- Anyone can walk for fitness. You need only a pair of properly fitting athletic shoes or walking boots, and somewhere to walk – a park, shopping centre or treadmill.
- Walking can be mild – where you can go on indefinitely; moderate – which can be sustained for up to 2 hours if you are already fairly fit, and you can talk easily; and race walking pace, which is high intensity and can be sustained for 30–45 minutes only by the already fit.

How long do you have to walk to burn fat?

Many in the exercise world believe that you should walk, or do other low intensity exercise, for only 20 minutes; exercising anything over and above that 20 minutes and you are only burning fat. This is a myth. Your body burns both glycogen (carbohydrate) and stored fat during exercise. Glycogen burning is favoured during the beginning of exercise and during intense exercise. Fat burning is maximised during sustained, low intensity exercise. The longer you work out the more exhausted, your supply of glycogen becomes and the more fat your body burns.

However, although you are burning more fat after 20 minutes, you are not only burning fat. The body always uses a combination of fat and carbohydrate during exercise.

Moderate-intensity, long duration (20–60 minutes) walking is for ideal fat loss. It is logical that the longer you walk, the more fat you will lose, and, if you get into a regular routine, you will maximise fat loss. But it is incorrect to think that there's a magic fat burning device that comes on after 20 minutes.

MBTs

I recommend MBT shoes because I've tried them, and I believe that they help you to exercise as you walk. MBTs claim to use the body's supporting muscle system when we are walking and standing upright. Conventional shoes support and lead the foot, stabilising the body in what they call an unnatural way. This means that these important muscles lose their function. Like any other inactive muscle, they atrophy, which can lead to joint and back pain. MBTs stimulate the body to balance itself by inducing a natural instability in the body which must constantly be compensated by the body's supporting muscle system. This natural instability underneath the feet ensures that neglected muscle groups automatically make the balancing movements that nature intended. These activated muscles relieve the pressure on joints and discs while walking. MBT have conducted clinical trials that support these claims. From my experience they help tone the legs, particularly hamstrings and buttocks. And anecdotal evidence suggests that they also help with joint and back pain. See resources for more details.

Strong women stay young

Morjorie

If there were a dictionary entry for 'anti-ageing' and how exercise can keep you youthful, a picture of Morjorie Newlin would be next to it. This mother of four, grandmother of four, and great grandmother of two is a staggering 87 years old (she was a sprightly 83 when the above picture was taken but says she looks better now!). Helen started working out in her late sixties to combat the aches and pains and loss of strength you experience as you get older (and are sedentary). She trains for 4 days per week, and her routine consists of strength training and 45 minutes of cardiovascular work, but she cuts down on the cardio if she starts to lose weight. She still competes in bodybuilding shows where she is well known on the natural bodybuilders circuit in America.

Morjorie says: 'I want to see women of all ages getting out there and working out. We only have one body and we have to honour it.' Wise words indeed Morjorie and we salute you. You too can incorporate the lifestyle changes outlined in the Programme that will ensure that you will be strong, firm and toned well into your eighties. Just like Morjorie.

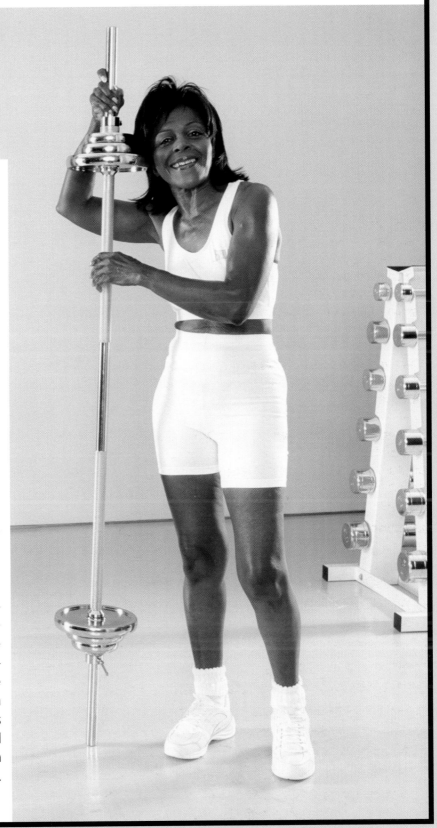

Stay strong,
Stay slim,
Look young!

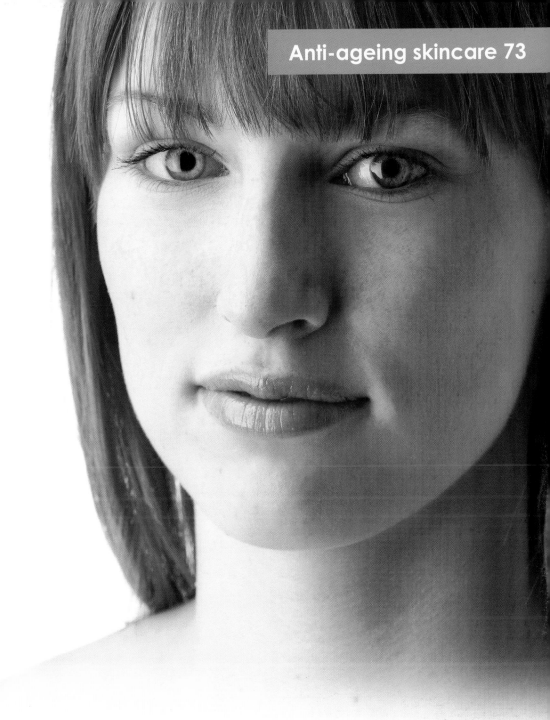

Chapter 4
Anti-ageing skincare

Anti-inflammatories
Peptides
Camelia oil
Antioxidants
Plant oils

What is it that turns our skin from the firm, dewy, supple skin of our youth, to the wrinkled, crêpey and puffy skin, complete with sagging jawline and jowls of our older years? Do we just need to accept this as part of getting older? The good news is no! Along with the other biomarkers included in the No Nips No Tucks Plan, aged skin can be prevented and to a degree, reversed, with simple lifestyle changes, without you having to revert to invasive cosmetic procedures and surgery.

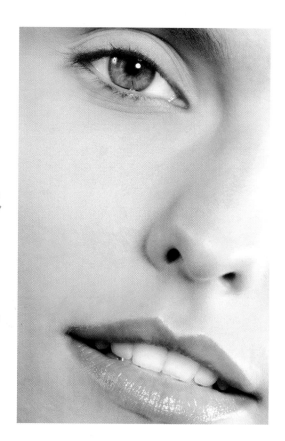

Why does skin age?

Skin ageing is principally caused by excessive free radical activity, which leads to inflammation.

The skin, as the outermost barrier of the body, is exposed to various sources of oxidative stress, in particular ultraviolet (UV) radiation and environmental toxins such as cigarette smoke, air pollution, etc. Internally, the skin is attacked like any other organ, through processes involving glycation (protein cross-linking), collagen–elastin degradation and free radical-induced injury.

One way of mitigating this process is to increase levels of protective antioxidants through a diet rich in fruits and vegetables, supplementation and by direct topical application. Indeed, various animal and human studies have proved that topically applied antioxidants exert protective effects against inflammation from free radical dam-

age. Free radicals form in skin upon UV exposure. Acute and chronic photo radiation damage depletes the body's natural antioxidant enzyme systems and increases oxidative protein modifications (cross-links). These pathological effects are found in the upper and lower layers of the skin. Cross-linked (glycated) proteins are classic characteristics of skin ageing. Cross-linked proteins in the skin result in stiffening, wrinkling and aged appearance.

As we discovered in the Eating section, glycation is a process that results in an abnormal bond between sugar and protein molecules and between protein molecules themselves. The end-products of glycation are called AGEs, or advanced glycation end-products, which attach to large proteins such as collagen, elastin, and other large molecules. You end up with a tired-looking puffy, doughy complexion with poor tone and wrinkled, leathery skin, but it can be turned around to restore the supple, glowing skin, high cheekbones and defined jawline.

I've already outlined the damage caused by glycation of collagen from the consumption of too many sugars and refined starches. High insulin levels, like sugar, are particularly damaging to our cells and cause increased free radicals, AGEs, and inflammation.

Too many sugars and refined carbohydrates in the diet also affect our ability to fight off infection. These processed foods do not come naturally packaged with the nutrients needed for them to be used as energy by the body. This means that they call on the body's reserves, depleting nutrients, which could be used for more crucial purposes, and affecting the immune system. Sugar also interferes with the way the body uses vitamin C, which is needed for the formation of collagen and elastin – necessary for healthy, supple skin, as well as for a strong immune system. Sugar and refined foods also create ideal conditions in the digestive tract for feeding yeasts and other unwanted organisms, which could lead to thrush or candida. It may also make your digestion sluggish, ultimately affecting all parts of the body, as well as your skin.

Environmental damage

The UV light that we receive from sunlight is a result of energy travelling in various wavelengths. The most damaging wavelength is called UV-B. Unfortunately for us, only a small percentage of this wavelength is absorbed by the ozone layer. UV radiation with a longer wavelength is called UV-A. These longer wavelengths are not considered quite as dangerous as UV-B. The vast majority of skin cancers are a result of UV-B. Our DNA and other large biological molecules absorb UV-B and UV-A, causing photo-damage and ageing.

Not enough oil

We've already mentioned the damage done to skin through low-fat diets. A sure way to dry out

your skin is to drastically reduce, or eliminate fat from your diet. Dry and/or ageing skin is characterised by a lack of oil and moisture caused by inadequate production of the sebaceous glands. In such cases the skin is out of balance and cannot be restored by external application of water-based creams. Water-based skin creams cannot penetrate the skin, and, in fact, even more moisture is taken from the surface of the skin through evaporation when water is applied.

Dry skin is more prone to forming wrinkles than any other skin type. Dry skin lacks softness, smoothness and suppleness. It feels tight, fragile and supersensitive. It cracks, flakes or peels. You moisturise it repeatedly with little or no results. Fine lines and wrinkles appear almost overnight. You look older than your years.

If these symptoms sound familiar, you're probably suffering from dry ageing skin. You're not alone. Millions of people are waging an ongoing battle against dry skin, which dermatologists and skin care specialists recognise as the most common complexion complaint.

With high hopes of restoring skin to its normal, moist and supple state, people may constantly feed their faces with the only weapons they know: creams, lotions and moisturisers. Despite vast amounts of cosmetics applied, your skin shows little change. Dry skin is usually a sign of an internal imbalance, and topical applied cosmetics alone cannot possibly correct a condition that originates internally.

Oil is very important to one's health, and it's very possible that many are suffering from problems that are directly attributable to insufficient oil. Your face shines from the inside out, and it is oil that makes that possible. Cook with healthful oils like extra virgin olive oil and coconut oil whenever possible. Have butter instead of low-fat spread and cream instead of low-fat synthetic substitutes. Oil is absolutely essential to obtaining the very best physical health.

Strong collagen

Collagen is a major structural protein in the skin. It plays a key role in providing the structural scaffolding for cells, tissues and organs. If it weren't for collagen, the body would literally fall apart. Collagen also gives the skin its strength and durability, and is responsible for the smooth, plump appearance of young, healthy skin. Understanding the structure and function of collagen will help you to know better how to maintain a healthy, youthful appearance.

What is collagen?

Collagen is the body's major structural protein composed of three protein chains wound together in a tight triple helix that gives collagen its unique tensile strength. Approximately 33% of the protein in the body is collagen. This protein supports tissues and organs and connects these structures to bones. Bones are also composed of collagen combined with certain minerals such as calcium and phosphorus.

Collagen makes up 75% of our skin; thus, the smooth, plump appearance of young, healthy skin is due in large part to the presence of healthy collagen levels. Because of this, any effective anti-ageing programme needs to boost collagen levels and repair past collagen damage – which this Programme aims to do. The breakdown of healthy collagen and the decline in collagen production leads to the development of unwanted wrinkles and the appearance of aged skin.

How is collagen made?

Collagen is created by fibroblasts, which are specialised skin cells located in the dermis. Fibroblasts also produce other skin structural proteins such as elastin (a protein which gives the skin its ability to snap back) and glucosaminoglycans (GAGs). GAGs make up the ground substance that keeps the dermis hydrated.

Vitamin C acts as a cofactor during the collagen-making process. Without sufficient levels of vitamin C, collagen formation is disrupted. Collagen synthesis occurs continuously throughout our lives to repair and replace damaged collagen tissue or build new cellular structures. The degradation and recycling of old or damaged collagen is a natural process used to create protein fragments needed to build new cellular structures, such as in the healing process.

The best way to maintain a healthy, youthful-looking appearance is to protect the healthy collagen you currently have and to prevent future collagen degradation. The are three main ways to do this are:
● avoid UVA and UVB radiation
● prevent free radical damage and inflammation
● prevent damage by glycation.

Exposure to ultraviolet (UV-A and UV-B) radiation emanating from the sun is the most prolific contributor to premature skin ageing, accounting for an estimated

90% of the signs associated with ageing skin. UV exposure must be limited and individuals should use products with sun filters and sun protection to protect healthy collagen.

The second preventive step in protecting existing and future collagen levels is supplementation with both oral and topical antioxidants. As antioxidants fight free radicals from UV light, ozone, pollution, cigarette smoke, and internal metabolic processes, they prevent the degradation of existing collagen fibres and protect the healthy function of fibroblast cells.

The third step is to balance blood sugar levels to avoid glycation and inflammation.

Promoting the synthesis of collagen

There are many ways to promote the synthesis of new, healthy collagen. First, you can provide the skin with a reserve of vitamin C. As a necessary co-factor in collagen synthesis, vitamin C is proven to increase the production of collagen. One study showed that extended exposure of human connective-tissue cells to vitamin C stimulated an 8-fold increase in the synthesis of collagen.

Secondly, collagen production can be boosted by supplementation. Silicon is an essential component of collagen and supplemental silicon increases the collagen content of the skin and cartilage. Also oral supplementation of collagen provides a way in which the body can be provided with vital amino acids and proteoglycans (specialised sugars in the body) important for the maintenance of connective tissues (see more in chapter on anti-ageing nutrients).

A third way to promote the synthesis of collagen is to exfoliate dead skin as consistent exfoliation stimulates cell renewal. Chemical exfoliation has also been shown to increase dermal thickness, which has been attributed to the synthesis of glycosaminoglycans and collagen within the dermis.

A fourth way to promote collagen synthesis is with collagen-stimulating peptides. Fibroblasts are naturally stimulated to begin the synthesis of collagen when specific combinations of peptide signal molecules (fibroblast growth factors) bind to receptor sites on the fibroblast membrane. These signal molecules can be applied topically to help boost collagen production, and are very effective when included in oil-based skincare products.

Oestrogen and skin ageing

Oestrogen appears to exert a strong influence on the ageing of the skin. Oestrogen receptors are located in the skin, and studies have shown that oestrogen increases the activity of skin fibroblasts, cells that produce collagen.

During the menopause, when the production of hormones in the ovaries diminishes significantly and eventually stops altogether, many women notice changes in their skin, most noticeably dryness and wrinkling. During the menopause the skin thins out and loses its elasticity causing wrinkles to deepen; the process of cell renewal slows down, resulting in less radiance and a duller complexion. Some estimates show that skin loses up to 30% of its collagen in the first 5 years after menopause, and without intervention, post-menopausal skin will continue to degenerate.

Maintaining optimal levels of oestrogen, however, appears to safeguard against many of these effects, and there are some very good books detailing natural alternatives to HRT, which has its dangers. Boosting levels of growth hormone naturally will also negate some of these effects.

Other enemies of beautiful skin

Alcohol in excess

Binge drinking and consuming high quantities of alcohol dehydrates the skin, leaving it dry and irritated. For people drinking more than 14 drinks a week, it can cause swollen blood vessels, resulting in tiny red veins to appear on the skin's surface making the face look flushed.

Smoking

This will age you – cut back or better yet cut it out altogether. It causes several adverse effects on skin. The nicotine from cigarettes narrows the blood vessels and prevents blood from circulating to the tiny blood vessels in the upper layer of the skin. This in course destroys collagen, with a smoker's skin characteristically having more, and deeper, wrinkles than non-smokers.

Lack of sleep

Getting enough sleep is important, because it is while we are sleeping that our body and skin has time to repair and rejuvenate.

Environmental pollution

City pollution as well as environmental factors such as air conditioning and central heating can all be harmful to our skin. Our skin can become coated in dirt from pollution, which blocks pores; alternate hot and cold from the air-con and heating can dry and then rehydrate the skin.

How to restore youthful skin

- Avoid refined carbohydrates and sugar to protect against inflammation and Glycation.
- Eat good fats.
- Protect collagen with antioxidants.
- Build collagen through diet and supplementation.
- Exfoliate frequently.
- Use effective topical applications containing peptides.
- Use sun protection.
- Supplement.

Use oil-based skincare

For many years, a debate raged in the dermatological community as to whether topically applied anti-ageing preparations could slow skin ageing. The scientific literature now indicates that the daily application of a variety of agents can have a profound effect on both the health and appearance of the skin.

Alpha-lipoic acid is a super-potent fat and water-soluble antioxidant, so it can protect the fat cells in the skin and cell membranes. It helps maintain the health of the mitochondria so skin cells can perform repair functions. In addition, alpha-lipoic acid helps turn off an inflammatory messenger known as nuclear factor kappa B (NFkB).The expression of NFkB induces inflammation at an early stage. Factors that suppress NFkB inhibit skin damaging inflammatory processes. Another benefit to having abundant quantities of alpha-lipoic acid in the skin is its ability to regulate a collagen-regulating factor known as AP-1. When alpha-lipoic acid activates AP-1, it turns on enzymes that digest only glycation-damaged collagen. In a study, high potency alpha-lipoic acid reduced mild-to-moderate wrinkles by up to 50%, whereas fine lines almost disappeared.

Today, mass market-oriented cosmetics manufacturers have replaced natural oils with less expensive synthetic ingredients. In contrast to delicate natural oils, for instance, a conventional moisturiser is likely to contain mineral oil, petroleum, detergents and animal fat by-products that can clog the pores causing further dryness and wrinkled skin.

Oils can be applied directly to the skin to nourish, soften and protect it. Certain oils can be used as a base in which essential oils are diluted. Oils are highly penetrating. They easily enter through a cell wall delivering essential vitamins, oxygen and nutrients. This helps to stimulate cell metabolism and cell regeneration. The ability of oils to penetrate and carry nutrients through the cell wall to the cell nucleus can prevent cell deterioration, which can lead to infections and diseases.

Many oils, such as coconut oil, have antibacterial properties thus helping to reduce infections in sensitive or damaged skin. Oils have been successfully used in skin care preparations for centuries. In the early 20th century, the cosmetics industry promoted the idea that oils were bad for the skin and it promoted the use of oil/water/detergent mixtures as moisturisers. The emulsions are considerably cheaper than using natural oils, though this fact is not always reflected in the price.

Oils also make very effective skin cleansers, and can remove make-up. The same mechanism works with everyday residues and impurities that accumulate on your skin. Oils effectively lift off the dirt, leaving the skin clean and nourished. Many oils, such as safflower oil, are rich in essential fatty acids. These acids preserve the protective function of cell membranes.

As stated earlier, inflammation is a major cause of skin ageing, and one of the most powerful anti-inflammatories that nature has provided is oleic acid, the primary fatty acid found in camellia oil. Camellia oil contains the highest amount of the monounsaturated fatty acid oleic acid in any cosmetic oil – over 82%. Oleic acid helps to keep the cell membrane soft and protects it against the inflammation that causes skin to age. It is a super-moisturiser that will make skin soft and supple.

We tested oleic acid rich Oleicia Facial Oils on women whose facial skin exhibited all of the physical signs of ageing, and some of the observations were that the oils:

● increased the skin's ability to retain moisture making it more supple and without making it greasy
● evened out skin colour
● increased skin's smoothness and radiance
● diminished fine lines, scarring and enlarged pores

On stretched tummies it also helped eliminate stretch marks and firmed the skin. Studies have demonstrated that oleic acid is capable of permeating deep into the lower layers of the stratum corneum of the skin. This ability to enhance permeation across the skin rejuvenates cell growth to give skin support and flexibility. Oleic acid is also an excellent transdermal carrier of nutrients into the skin to repair the damage caused by environmental pollution, sun and other factors. This increased permeation will improve the skin's elasticity, resulting in more youthful, supple and resilient skin, and reducing or eliminating fine lines and wrinkles.

Oleic acid is the main fatty acid produced by the skin's sebaceous glands and is very similar in nature and pH to sebum, the oil naturally secreted by the sebaceous glands. Sebum protects and moisturises the skin and hair, but is stripped away by chemicals, pollutants, the sun and age, resulting in dry skin and hair. Oleic acid-based products replenishes what our skin and hair loses, and restores their natural balance without clogging pores.

For details of where you can find Oleicia products, and other effective products for ageing skin see resources on page 138.

Chapter 5
Anti-ageing haircare

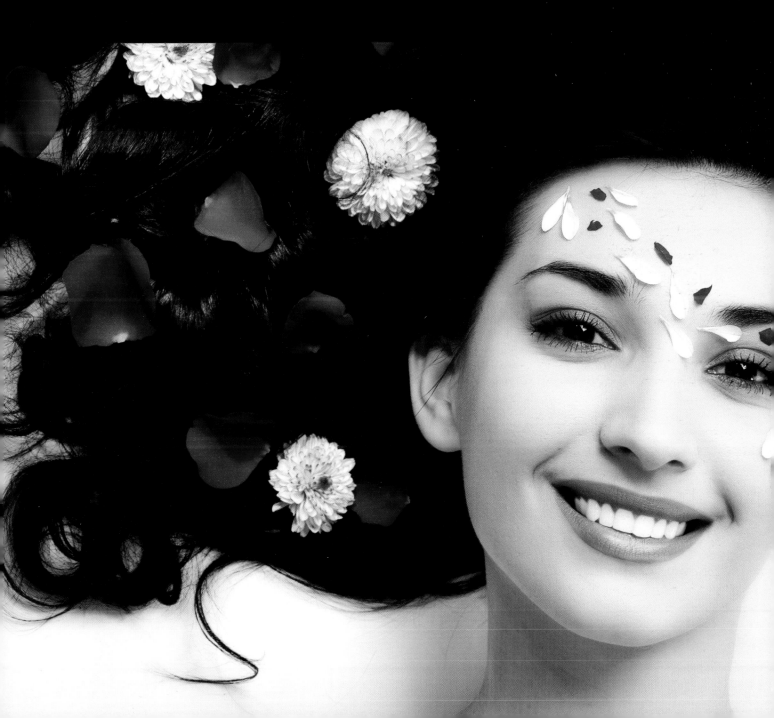

Amino acids
Fleeceflower
MSM
Collagen

As we age, our hair also ages. The volume of hair can decrease, and also the strength, thickness and longevity of each hair follicle can also diminish. However, there are steps that you can take that can prevent further hair thinning and loss, while increasing the strength, health, and diameter of the hair follicle.

After years of abuse from perms, bleaches, braids, weaves, extensions and many more processes, it's inevitable that hair will suffer. As far as professional advice goes, drugs, or a hair transplant are the only available solution to problems of hair loss. That's good for the pharmaceutical companies and transplant surgeons, but many are unaware that there are proven natural alternatives.

That's where the bad news ends and the good news starts. If your hair has suffered as you've aged, there is a lot that you can do about it. A good understanding of how and why certain things work can be life changing – and in order to turn things around, it is important to have at least a fundamental understanding of how and why hair loss occurs.

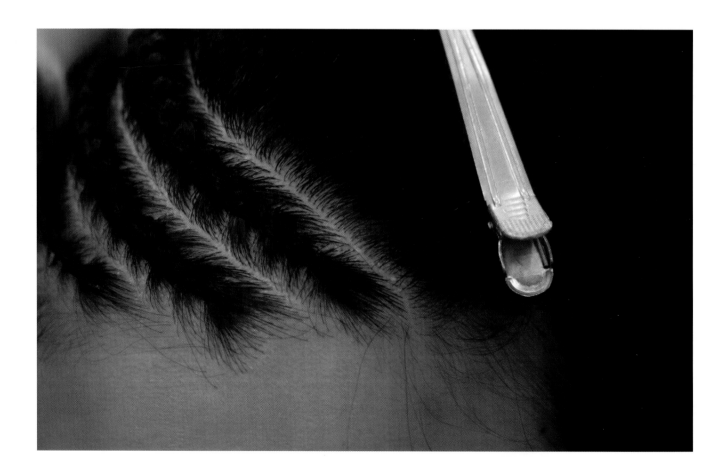

How hair grows

The structure of the hair follicle is protein. There are eight amino acids that the body does not produce and which therefore must come from complete protein foods such as eggs, dairy (milk, cheese, yogurt, etc.), meat, fish, and fowl. Eat some protein at each meal.

Hair growth isn't a constant – it grows in cycles. The growth cycle (anagen phase) lasts several years followed by a resting cycle. The final result is a fall-out cycle. A full, thick head of hair is due to a rate of hair growth that is greater or equal than the fall-out. When the growth cycle begins to slow down your hair begins to recede; hair strands become thin in appearance, and shortly after, fall out (catagen stage).

The rest phase (telegen phase) lasts about 2–6 months, the growth period continues for 2–6 years. During the on and off again activity, about 50–100 hairs per day fall out.

Why do follicles eventually stop making hair altogether and leave us bald? Often lack of blood flow to the hair follicle stifles hair production, this suppresses the follicle productivity and thin hair results.

Preventing grey hair

Fleeceflower
A Chinese herb called ho-shou-wu (fleeceflower or fo-ti root: Polygonum multiflorum) is very effective in maximising hair growth stages for the benefit of hair preservation. The literal English translation for ho-shou-wu is 'black hair Mr. He', which speaks for its ability to preserve natural hair colour, and turn hair from grey to its original colour, which is one of the benefits of long time usage.

As previously mentioned, a full, thick head of hair is due to a rate of hair growth that is greater or equal than the fall-out. Fleeceflower prolongs the anagen phase or growth cycle, while minimising the resting (telegen) and fall-out (catagen) stages.

Chinese medical theories believe that your hair's condition is an indication of your body's internal system. Weaknesses in a person's kidney and liver tend to manifest into symptoms such as hair loss and premature grey hair. A study was conducted in China, testing fo-ti root to see if it would increase circulation and lower blood cholesterol in elderly patients. During the studies with the herb, an interesting side effect was noted: The patient's hair began to return to its natural colour, and became thicker and shinier.

At the Hospital of Prevention and Therapeutics/Chemical Industry Shashi Hubei, China, a study was performed on 882 patients for the treatment of hair loss.[1] Each received a preparation of fo-ti root for 3 months. Of those patients, 630 were cured. Only 48 patients did not respond at all. Additional benefits revealed a reduction of serum cholesterol levels.

Fo-ti root is also thought to be a tonic for the endocrine glands, liver and kidneys. Fo-ti root contains many vitamins and minerals that are vital for hair, specifically the B-complex vitamins, vitamin C, silicon, zinc and Vitamin A.[2, 3]

Controlling superoxides

A chronic type of inflammation at the site of the hair follicle can suppress hair growth. This is much like an allergic response from an overactive immune system. Hair cells can be treated by our immune system as a foreign body. An immunological attack to the hair follicle is from the inflammation of the blood vessels that feed the hair follicle. The actual reason for this isn't completely understood; however, it is known that controlling a damaging substance called superoxide can help stop this inflammation.

When a follicle bulb atrophies, in large part it is due from the attack of superoxide. This is what causes follicle miniaturisation and ultimately the loss of hair. Too much superoxide can limit the body's supply of nitric oxide, which is vital for blood flow through the capillaries that feed hair follicles.

Eating a regular diet of cooked, processed food and little to none of raw, whole, unrefined foods contributes to excess occupation of the superoxide free radical. Too much superoxide is destined to increase inflammation, specifically the capillaries that supply hair follicles with nutrients.

A proteolytic enzyme bromelain, glucosamine sulphate and MSM are all anti-inflammatory substances that can also benefit your joints as well as your hair.

Whole, unprocessed foods normally contain the antioxidants needed to control the superoxide that helps aggravate inflammation in the scalp. Superoxide can be broken down by the enzyme superoxide dismutase (SOD); a powerful antioxidant manufactured by the body and obtained from whole food sources. Abundant amounts of SOD are found in wheat grass and barley green.

Ageing minimises the body's ability to withstand the damage from superoxide because enzymes like superoxide dismutase are not as prevalent in our bodies as we get older.

Human growth hormone also stimulates hair growth on newly balding areas (see page 97 for natural ways to boost HGH).

Amino acids and MSM

Amino acids are what the cell uses to make protein, and it has been found that amino acid balances are inadequate in individuals with poor hair. The body can manufacture all but eight of the amino acids. These eight amino acids are considered essential to health and must be obtained from outside sources, like food or supplements. Without amino acids, cells cannot maintain or repair themselves. Protein deficiency, even short-term, results in dramatic changes in the hair roots. These changes include a reduction in hair diameter, and weaker hair.

The most important amino acids for the health of your hair are:
● L-cysteine and L-methionine. These two amino acids improve quality, texture and growth of hair. Cysteine is present in alpha-keratin, the chief protein in hair. Methionine helps prevent brittle hair. The synthesis of the amino acid cysteine may be dependent on the availability of methionine. Lecithin is a good source of methionine as well as inositol.

● L-arginine. Another amino acid good for hair. It is the metabolic precursor for nitric oxide, which is a messenger substance that stimulates hair growth by opening potassium channels. It also enhances sexual performance.

● Methylsulphonylmethane (MSM) is a vital supplement to improve hair condition. It plays a major role in the structural maintenance of the scalp capillaries. MSM contains both amino acids cysteine and methionine, and has a host of benefits besides assisting hair growth. MSM will help hair grow as fast as it is able. It is also an effective anti-inflammatory.

Minerals

When copper is converted to its organic form by binding to peptides (small fragments of proteins), it can be safely applied to the skin. Such copper peptides have been shown to promote collagen synthesis and thereby stimulate hair growth, as well as skin healing.

The mineral silica has been shown to support the structure of blood vessel walls that supply nutrients to follicle hair roots.

Zinc is another mineral that should be considered essential. It can help to combat superoxide, the principal precursor of many other free radicals. Zinc; along with copper help with the destruction of superoxide.

Vitamins

Since a dynamic blood supply is necessary for keeping hair follicles productive, the B-vitamins, including niacin, thiamine and biotin, can enhance hair health by improving factors that promote circulation of blood to the skin of the scalp.

Essential fatty acids

Finally essential fatty acids (EFAs) help improve hair texture and prevent dry, brittle hair. Omega-3 is the most important, and this is the most deficient one in our diet. Gamma-linolenic acid (GLA), an omega-6 fatty acid found in unrefined evening primrose oil, hemp seed and blackcurrant oils are very beneficial as well.

As with skin, oleic acid from camellia oil can benefit hair by helping prevent the oxidation of keratin protein when applied to the hair, resulting in soft, lustrous and shiny hair.

Male pattern baldness is a hereditary condition that most often affects men, but may affect women as well. Although the exact reason for the hair loss is not clear, some studies suggest that excessive conversion of testosterone to another hormone called dihydrotestosterone (DHT) may be an underlying cause.

Saw palmetto

The herb Saw palmetto and beta-sitosterol (which is found in Saw palmetto) have been shown to block the production of dihydrotestosterone (DHT) in men suffering from enlargement of the prostate, and high levels of DHT is also implicated with male pattern baldness. And studies have shown that these compounds also help with hair loss, without causing significant side effects.

These findings are encouraging for millions of men (and possibly women) with male pattern hair loss. Women of childbearing age should take caution though because Saw Palmetto has not been proven to be safe during pregnancy and lactation.

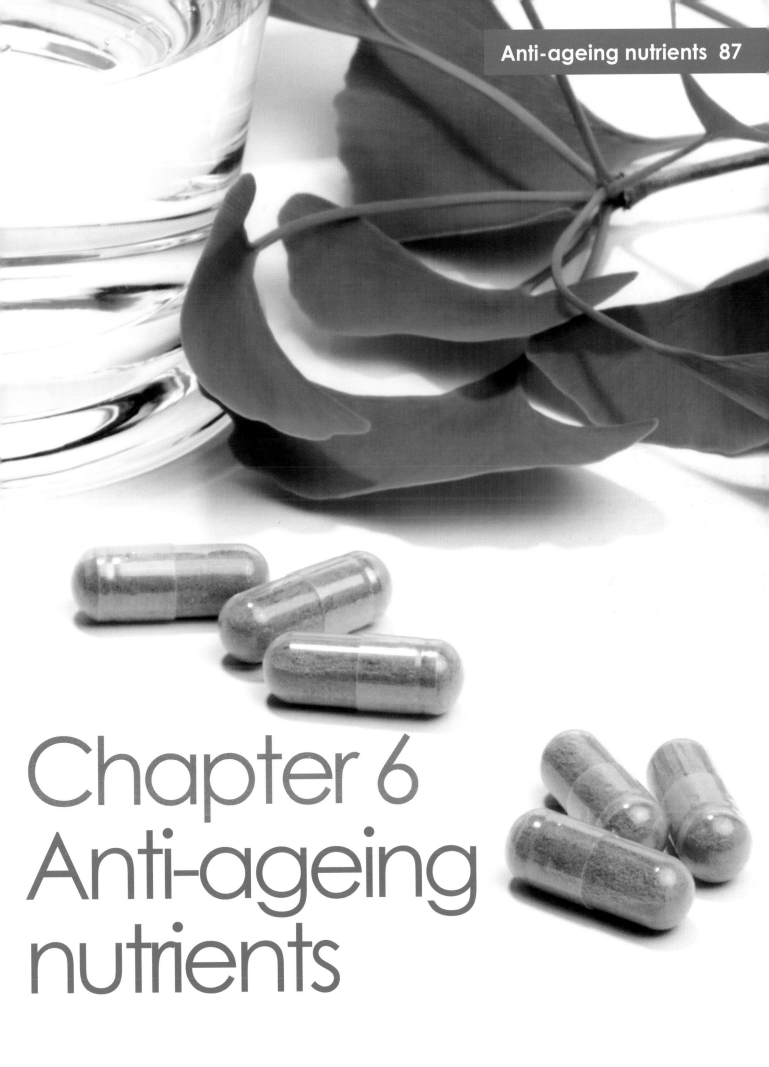

Chapter 6
Anti-ageing
nutrients

Alpha-lipioc acid
Co-enzyme Q10
Collagen
Enzymes & Probiotics

Why supplement?

There are some very good reasons why we need to supplement our diets, and especially an anti-ageing diet. The first and most important reason is that the nutrients required by the body to help slow down and reverse ageing are simply not in the foods we eat in sufficient quantities to make any significant difference. We couldn't possibly eat the amount of food it takes to get those nutrients. There are also other important reasons:

The toxic load on our bodies from chemicals including pesticides and pollution means that our bodies need an optimum supply of nutrients to combat their effects.
The nutrients that we need are no longer found in the soil in rich supply because of intensive farming, so they won't be in plants or animals.

Also, various stressors such as illness, injury, inflammation and stress deplete the body's store of nutrients needed to combat ageing, and can stimulate the release of stress hormones such as adrenalin.

Anti-ageing effects of supplements

To be effective against ageing, supplements will need to be able to perform either or all of these three functions:

A. exerting protective effects against free radical induced inflammation
B. exerting protective effects against glycation
C. protecting, or increasing the body's production of collagen.

On the following pages appears a review of the scientific studies and clinical trials on the effectiveness of the nutrients that have been shown to have an anti-ageing effect. Based on this research, we have formulated two supplements, one – Protective Nutrients – is a blend of antioxidants and other nutrients that have been shown to protect cells from free radical damage, and to repair and regenerate cells. The other – Skin, Hair and Nails Formula – contains nutrients that have been shown to be essential for healthy and youthful skin, hair and nails. See resources for details.

Alpha-lipoic acid – protective effects: A & B

Alpha-lipoic acid is an important antioxidant that is both fat soluble and water soluble enabling it to provide antioxidant protection of the cell membrane where it is believed much free-radical damage takes place.

It facilitates the production of energy for cells and enhances the effectiveness of other antioxidants.[1] Studies have shown that it can reactivate vitamin C from its oxidised form, and studies have also shown that it can reactivate vitamin E.

Alpha-lipoic acid can enhance the synthesis of glutathione, the main antioxidant within our cells.[2, 3] Glutathione effectively mops up all types of toxins and free radicals. However, we cannot take supplements of this antioxidant since it is unable to cross cell membranes; therefore one has to rely on substances that enhance its synthesis. Fortunately, both laboratory and animal studies have shown that alpha-lipoic acid can stimulate the production of glutathione.

It may help the body establish more healthy blood sugar levels while treating some of the neurological side effects diabetes,[4] and may help to prevent the development of hyperglycaemia. According to a study published in 1997, alpha-lipoic acid was found to reduce glycation of proteins in human tissues.

In combination with acetyl-L-carnitine it can reduce signs of lipid peroxidation and improve memory.[5]

Usage
Low doses of alpha-lipoic acid, such as 10–50 mg, do not cause side effects of any significance. Higher doses of 200 mg or more per day could cause gastrointestinal symptoms of nausea or stomach upset.

Acetyl-L-carnitine – protective effects: A

Acetyl-L-carnitine (ALC) is a chemical product of the amino acid, carnitine. It is produced naturally in humans, with the greatest amounts being found in muscles, the brain and testicles. ALC has been studied for its potential use in slowing, and even partially reversing, nerve and brain deterioration associated with the ageing process.

As part of its role in supporting mental function, ALC may improve memory, attention span, and mental performance in normal people as well as those with brain impairment. Acetyl-L-carnitine readily crosses the blood–brain barrier[6] and thus confers powerful protective effects on nerve tissue and the central nervous system – enhancing mood, restoring energy and alleviating nerve pain.

It is also instrumental in the production and release of one of the brain's vital neurotransmitters, acetylcholine. ALC may also support healthy function of the male reproductive system and improve intracellular energy transfer.

ALC has been studied for its potential use in treating a number of disorders. Some studies have demonstrated memory improvement when participants were given the combination of ALC and lipoic acid. Studies suggest that ALC can slow the progression of Alzheimer's disease.[7]

Usage
500–1000 mg per day.

Coenzyme Q10 – protective effects: A

Coenzyme Q10 (Co-Q10) is an important vitamin-like compound that is present throughout the body. While there are 10 other coenzyme Q compounds present in nature, Co-Q10 is the only one present in humans.

Co-Q10's benefits are due to the following two attributes.

● It is an important fat-soluble antioxidant that is uniquely able to protect the cells' energy-producing machinery, the mitochondria, from free radical damage.
● It is necessary for the production of energy in all cells of the body.

Co-Q10 is incorporated into the mitochondria of cells throughout the body where it facilitates and regulates the transformation of fats and sugars into energy. A large body of scientific evidence shows that Co-Q10's ability to restore mitochondrial function has a profound effect on one's overall health.[8]

An important application for Co-Q10 is in the treatment and prevention of cardiovascular disease and related disorders that involve the heart, including atherosclerosis.[9–14] Studies have suggested that Co-Q10 can reduce the frequency of angina episodes, strengthen the heart muscle and increase quality of life and survivability in those with congestive heart failure. Co-Q10 has also been shown to decrease blood pressure in patients with high blood pressure.

Of potential benefit to diabetics is the fact that Co-Q10 may enhance insulin production. Also, obesity may also be linked to a deficiency of Co-Q10. Studies have suggested that supplementation can enhance weight loss and it has been suggested that Co-Q10 could be beneficial in the treatment of patients with chronic fatigue syndrome.

Levels of Co-Q10 decline with age. Studies on ageing showed an average 57% reduction in Co-Q10 levels in seven different tissues in the body.[15–19]

Usage

Supplement recommendation is at least 100 mg of regular Co-Q10 each day. Higher intakes of CoQ10 could produce greater benefits.[20]

Green tea extract – protective effects: A & B

Green tea is one of nature's most potent agents in protecting the body against a host of illnesses.

Research conducted in the last few years suggests that it may be effective in helping to prevent a wide variety of cancers in humans, including cancers of the bladder, colon, oesophagus, pancreas, rectum and stomach.

The active ingredients in green tea thought to be principally responsible for chemoprevention are polyphenols, the natural antioxidant compounds found in plants. Tea contains four main polyphenols called catechins, which are water-soluble compounds making up a subgroup of flavonoids, also commonly found in fruits and vegetables, coffee, chocolate, and wine. Catechins are powerful antioxidants that can be easily oxidised in the body; their antioxidant potential has been found to be significantly higher than that of grape juice and red wine.

The catechins present in green tea include epigallocatechin-3 gallate (EGCG), epigallocatechin (EGC), and epicatechin-3 gallate (ECG).

A study of heart disease risk in men showed that a higher dietary intake of flavonoids, primarily from tea, was associated with decreased mortality from coronary heart disease. and a decreased incidence of myocardial infarction, or heart attack.[21]

Green tea may also slow the effects of normal ageing and its associated decline in brain function. A 2004 study investigated the effect of long-term green tea catechin intake on ageing and oxidative damage, using aged mice with cerebral atrophy and cognitive dysfunction. Catechin intake was shown to effectively suppress further atrophy and cognitive dysfunction,[22] strongly suggesting that green tea can at least partially improve the negative functional changes that occur naturally in ageing brains.

Epidemiological data suggest that green tea consumption prevents type 2 diabetes and promotes healthy glucose metabolism.[23] In healthy human volunteers, green tea promoted healthy glucose metabolism, as determined by oral glucose tolerance tests. Green tea also lowered blood glucose levels in diabetic mice without affecting serum insulin levels. Green tea therefore appears to have antihyperglycaemic effects.

Usage
Around 200 mg per day.

Grapeseed extract – protective effects: A & C

Oligomeric proanthocyanidins (OPCs) are found in many woody plants. The two most common sources of OPCs are grape seeds (Vitis vinifera) and the white pine (Pinus maritima, P. pinaster) of southern Europe. Grape seeds can have 7–15% more OPCs than pine bark and can be more potent as well as more economical.[24]

An animal study found that a patented grape seed extract protected tissue from oxidation better than the antioxidant vitamins C and E or beta-carotene.[25]

Oxidised low-density lipoproteins (LDL) damage the cells that line blood vessel walls by provoking numerous responses including inflammation, smooth muscle cell proliferation and clotting mechanisms, all of which lead to atherosclerosis. A grape seed extract with 50% OPCs and 50% phenolic acids prevented such oxidation of pig LDL in vitro.[26]

In vitro studies suggest that OPCs provide cancer protection. A study found that a patented grape seed extract killed cancer cells; inhibited growth of human breast, lung, stomach and myelogenous leukaemia cells by up to 73%; and enhanced normal cell growth.[27]

Collagen is an important factor in providing structure and strength of the skin. OPCs have an affinity for connective tissue components, such as collagen, and human studies have shown that OPCs protect against the effects of certain enzymes that 'digest' and weaken collagen and elastin. Collagen and elastin appear to be reinforced by OPCs. Thus, OPCs may help protect collagen and elastin.

Part of the ageing process is the degradation of skin by the enzyme elastase, which is released with the inflammatory response. OPCs specifically block elastase, thus maintaining the integrity of elastin.[28]

OPCs can also reduce reddening of the skin by 13%. A study looked at the effect of an OPC dietary supplement on skin reddening (erythema) induced by exposure to UV radiation. The researchers report that while the formulations did reduce skin reddening, the people receiving the dietary supplement of OPCs had 13% less erythema than those receiving no supplement. Levels of skin hydration were also said to be higher in the group taking the dietary supplement.

Usage

100 mg extract per day (equivalent to dry seed 12 g).

Beta-carotene – protective effects: A

Beta-carotene is a substance from plants that the body converts into vitamin A. It is one of nearly 600 different chemicals known as carotenoids or carotenes, substances that give fruits and vegetables an orange colour. While vitamin A can be toxic if taken in amounts greater than needed by the body, beta-carotene can be safely ingested even in large quantities.

Like vitamin A, beta-carotene is a powerful antioxidant, though the disease-fighting power of this and other carotenes appears to be of greatest value when it is derived from foods rather than supplements.

Food sources of beta-carotene include dark leafy greens, carrots, sweet potatoes, pumpkin, apricots and broccoli.

Usage
1.6–60 mg per day.

Silicon – protective effects: C

Silica is an essential nutrient for strong and healthy skin, hair and nails. Blood vessels, bone, cartilage, hair, nails and skin are all composed wholly or partially of connective tissue, made up of proteins (e.g. collagen, elastin) and protein-sugar complexes such as chondroitin sulphate. Silicon is concentrated in the connective tissue and is thought to play a role in cross-linking connective tissue structures, thereby helping to create their tough, but flexible strength. A lack of silicon is known to reduce normal growth and repair of the skin, hair and nails.[29]

Sources of silica include: horsetail; bamboo (tabashir, also spelled tabasheer and tabaschir, a pearl opal organic stone); algae; colloidal silicon; silicon enriched yeast; choline stabilised orthosilicic acid.

Orthosilicic acid, which consists of only one silicon atom bonded to four hydroxides instead of oxygen, is the form of silicon that is found in our bloodstream.

Bamboo is the richest known source of natural silica containing over 70% organic silica. The abundance of silica in bamboo causes a silica gel to form in the hollow stem of the plant called tabashir. This is more than 30 times the level found in the horsetail plant (Equisetum), which contains about 2–3% silica. The bamboo extract is prepared from tabashir bamboo stem (Bambusa vulgaris). Bamboo is consumed in Asia, where it is known for its healthful properties.

Silicon is important for optimal collagen synthesis and is crucial for activating the hydroxylation enzymes for cross-linking collagen, which improves its strength and elasticity. Stronger collagen means better skin, more elasticity and fewer wrinkles.

The outer shaft of hair, that provides elasticity and strength, is rich in silicon. Hair with higher silicon content tends to fall out less and has more shine and lustre. Silicon is one of the predominant minerals in nails. A sign that silicon may be systematically deficient is brittle and soft nails. Silicon improves the nail quality resulting in a better protection against nail infections. Studies have shown that silicon makes hair and nails grow faster, stronger and in the case of hair, thicker by up to 49%.[30, 31]

Silicon also has an effect on joints, tendons and ligaments by formation of articular cartilage. It is also a cross-linking agent in the glycosaminoglycan network, which attracts and holds water in the joint. The activity of prolylhydroxylase, a specific enzyme for collagen synthesis, was shown to be silicon dependent in vitro.

Usage 100 mg daily.

Collagen – protective effects: C

Oral supplementation of collagen provides a way in which the body can be provided with vital amino acids and proteoglycans (specialised sugars in the body), important for maintenance of connective tissues, and replacing lost collagen.

Collagen type I and III are the chief collagen types in hair, skin, nails, tendons, ligament, muscles, bones, teeth, eyes and blood vessels. Although their presence is beneficial in joint tissues, collagen type II is the true major component of joint cartilage. Collagen type II (particularly from chicken sternal cartilage) supplies vital amino acids, hyaluronic acid, chondroitin and glucosamine for optimal joint cartilage support.

There is no clinical evidence that collagen supplements lead to either firmer skin or weight loss; however, there is plenty of anecdotal evidence that people who have taken collagen have reported that their skin became firmer and more supple, hair grows thicker and nails grow faster and less brittle.

Usage
6 g daily.

Vitamin E – protective effects: A

Vitamin E is a fat-soluble antioxidant that fights damaging free radicals. It works in lipids (fats and oils), making it complementary to vitamin C, which fights free radicals dissolved in water.

As an antioxidant, vitamin E has been widely advocated for preventing heart disease and cancer. However, the results of large, well-designed trials have generally not been encouraging.

Usage
15 mg per day equals 22 international units (IU) natural vitamin E (22 IU X 0.67 = 15 mg) or 33 IU synthetic vitamin E (33 IU X 0.45 = 15 mg).

Vitamin C – protective effects: A & C

Vitamin C is a water-soluble vitamin that has a number of biological functions. Acting as an antioxidant, one of vitamin C's important functions is to protect LDL cholesterol from oxidative damage. (Only when LDL is damaged does cholesterol appear to lead to heart disease, and vitamin C may be one of the most important antioxidant protectors of LDL).[32] Vitamin C may also protect against heart disease by reducing the stiffness of arteries and the tendency of platelets to clump together.[33]

Vitamin C is needed to make collagen, the 'glue' that strengthens many parts of the body, such as muscles, blood vessels and skin. Vitamin C also plays important roles in wound healing and as a natural antihistamine.

Ascorbyl palmitate is a fat-soluble vitamin C prepared from ascorbic acid with palmitic acid. Since this form of vitamin C is fat soluble, it is stored in the lipid cell membrane until the body is ready to put it to use, therefore extending its availability to the cells unlike the water-soluble form. Ascorbyl palmitate protects the cell membranes in the skin, and water-soluble ascorbic acid protects the cytosol, the watery interior of the cell.

Usage
Some scientists have recommended that healthy people take large amounts of vitamin C for the prevention of illness. However, little or no research supports this point of view and it remains controversial. Supplementing more results in an excretion level virtually identical to intake, meaning that consuming more vitamin C does not increase the amount that remains in the body.[34] For cosmetic purposes 500 mg per day is recommended.

Because ascorbyl palmitate can be stored in the body's fat stores, intake should not exceed 500 mg per day.

Glucosamine sulphate – protective effects: C

A randomised, controlled study was conducted with 53 female volunteers who were supplied with an oral supplement containing glucosamine, amino acids, minerals and various antioxidant compounds. Hydration properties of the skin as well as textural analysis of the women's fine lines and wrinkles were assessed following 5 weeks' intake of the oral supplement with results compared with those of a control group of 12 people who did not take the supplement.

The results showed a statistically significant reduction in the number of visible wrinkles and a reduction in the number of fine lines in the group of women who took the supplement.[35] It did not, however, affect epidermal hydration.

Usage
400 mg daily

L-glutamine – protective effects: A

L-glutamine is the most prevalent amino acid in the blood. Human cells readily manufacture L-glutamine and under normal circumstances, dietary intake and production of L-glutamine is sufficient. However, in times of stress or increased energy output, the body's tissues need more L-glutamine than usual, making supplementation important.

L-glutamine can be found in beans, brewer's yeast, brown rice bran, dairy products, eggs, fish, legumes, meat, nuts, seafood, seeds, soy, whey, whole grains and beet root.

One of L-glutamine's most important functions involves the support of cellular energy, growth and repair.

Usage
1500 mg daily

N-acetyl cysteine (NAC) – protective effects: A

NAC, derived from the simple amino acid cysteine, provides significant protection against a broad array of modern toxins including acrolein (found in cigarette smoke and car exhaust). Research indicates that in addition to providing toxin protection, NAC is a selective immune system enhancer, improving symptoms and preventing recurrences of common lung-related illnesses such as chronic bronchitis.[36] NAC helps the body convert and synthesise glutathione, an amino acid compound that consists of glycine, L-glutamic acid and L-cysteine, and is found in every cell. While glycine and L-glutamic acid are plentiful in our diets, the amount of glutathione our bodies can produce is limited by their store of cysteine, which is sometimes in short supply. Supplementation with NAC thus helps the body produce glutathione at more beneficial levels.

NAC does not occur in foods. Its precursor, L-cysteine, occurs in most high-protein foods.

Usage

While cysteine, the amino acid from which N-acetyl cysteine is derived, is found in most high-protein foods, N-acetyl cysteine is not derived from dietary sources. Optimal levels of supplementation are uncertain, but a considerable proportion of the research studies on N-acetyl cysteine used 250–1500 mg per day.

Methyl sulphonyl methane (MSM) – protective effects: A

MSM is a natural sulphur-containing compound that is produced in the human body. Although MSM occurs naturally in foods, even moderate food processing destroys most of it. It provides an important source of sulphur, which plants, animals and humans need for a wide variety of processes. Biological sulphur is a major component in many of the body's proteins, tissues, hormones and enzymes.

Because MSM can inhibit pain impulses, promote blood flow, and reduce inflammation of tissues, it has also been researched for use as a pain reliever and anti-inflammatory treatment. MSM has been researched for its ability to reduce pain associated with a long list of disorders.

Trace amounts of MSM occur in meats, fruits, and vegetables.

When applied topically, MSM may also reduce scarring and provide benefit for people with scleroderma, a disorder that involves hardening of the skin.

Usage

1 g per day.

Dimethylaminoethanol (DMAE) – protective effects: A

DMAE is a naturally occurring substance found in the flesh of fish, especially salmon. Animal studies show that taking DMAE results in increased levels of choline in the blood and brain. The increased levels of choline, in theory, should increase the body's ability to make acetylcholine, a very important neurotransmitter in the brain. Acetylcholine is involved in memory, learning, recall, and thought processes.

Internally, DMAE is a potent, site-specific free radical scavenger.[37] Taken in the proper dosage, DMAE's antioxidant effects can offer probable benefits in the maintenance of overall cellular health.

Usage

250 mg per day.

Other products

Growth hormone Secretagogues

Growth hormone secretagogues can cause the pituitary gland to release growth hormone, which declines as we get older. Numerous nutrients can acts as secretagogues, including amino acids such as glutamine, lysine, and arginine, and rather than injecting hGH which is expensive and carries some risks, GH secretagogues are perhaps the best alternative to naturally increase growth hormone levels.

Symbiotropin

It has been argued that human growth hormone (hGH) holds the key to the ageing process. Studies have shown that signs of ageing can be reversed by injections of hGH. Further studies investigated the body's mechanisms for producing hGH, and it was discovered that the production of the hormone does not decline with age – the body continues to produce hGH. What actually declines is the body's efficiency in releasing the hormone that it is still producing. They identified substances called secretagogues, which enhance the body's production, release and use of the hormone.

In clinical trials, participants taking the growth hormone secretagogue symbiotropin showed lost body fat, increased lean tissue, thicker skin, reduced wrinkles, thicker hair and restoration of its original colour, increased energy, improved sleep, plus many other changes.[38]

Amino acids

An amino acid called gamma-aminobutyric acid (GABA) has been shown to help increase HGH when taken internally. You can enjoy the benefits of hGH without paying a high price. GABA is a gamma-neurotransmitter. It's high in concentration in the hypothalamus, so it plays a significant role in hypothalamic-pituitary function. The pituitary gland is the master endocrine gland affecting all hormonal functions of the body including growth hormone. The hypothalamus is a region of the posterior section of the brain and is the regulating centre for visceral (instinctive) functions, such as sleep cycles, body temperature, and the activity of the pituitary gland.

There have been literally hundreds of clinical studies on GABA and numerous studies on GABA's ability to elevate growth hormone levels. A study from the First Medical Clinic at the University of Milan, Italy, stated: 'In all of the 19 subjects studied, compared with 18 controls, plasma growth hormone levels were significantly increased (above 5 mg/ml) by acute oral administration of 5g of GABA'.

Another study showed over a 5 1/2-fold increase in plasma growth hormone levels 90 minutes after GABA administration – a significant increase. GABA's growth hormone-elevating effects is said to rival that of potent pharmaceutical compounds.

Certain other amino acids (arginine, lysine and ornithine) can promote the body's natural release of growth hormone. Arginine and lysine are essential amino acids and therefore have to be derived from the food we eat. It has been shown in studies that ingestion of 1.5g of arginine will increase human growth hormone (hGH) secretion by blocking release of the hGH-inhibitor somatostatin, although some studies have suggested this causes gastric disturbance. However, 2g of glutamine will lead to elevation of human growth hormone (hGH) 90 minutes later without side effects. It may also be a good idea to ingest some amino acids after exercise, as this has been shown to enhance human growth hormone (hGH) secretion too.

Ornithine is non-essential and the body can make it, therefore supplementation is not as necessary. Proper medical supervision by a doctor is required in supplementing these compounds, since the glutamine-arginine-lysine stack may release insulin as well as growth hormone.

Enzymes and Probiotics

Enzymes

Digestive enzymes are complex molecules produced by both plants and animals designed to break down food components into smaller molecules. These small molecules can then be absorbed into the body either for recombination into new structures in the body (e.g. proteins for muscles) or to act as fuel for the body. They are produced internally from specialised organs in the body, or are derived externally from raw, unprocessed food. Cooking and food processing destroys virtually all enzymes in raw food.

Much of the raw food we do eat contains low levels of enzymes due to depleted soils, pollution, storage and preservation techniques (e.g. pasteurisation), and cooking. A low level of enzymes from external sources means more have to be produced internally, leading to over-burdening of the digestive system and the body's enzyme-producing capacity. An over-stressed digestion can lead to poor nutrient absorption, chronic fatigue, and digestive upset (bloating, pain, constipation etc.) Partially digested food can cross the gut wall and trigger the immune system, leading to an inflammatory situation in the body which can contribute to allergy syndromes and degenerative disease. An immune system having to constantly support the digestive system is limited in its ability to carry out its function of fighting disease and infection.

We also tend to produce fewer enzymes as we get older, it is therefore wise to occasionally supplement the diet with a digestive enzyme blend.

Probiotics

Probiotics are the beneficial bacteria that are absolutely essential for proper digestion, strong immune function and overall good health. They play an especially important role in keeping in check the pathogenic bacteria that cause disease. While it's true that non-beneficial bacteria are naturally occurring in the intestinal tract, problems begin when their growth goes unchecked.

When the ratio of good bacteria to bad is lowered problems arise such as excessive gas, bloating, intestinal toxicity, constipation and poor absorption of nutrients. A healthy lower intestine should contain at least 85% friendly bacteria to prevent the over colonisation of disease causing microorganisms like E. coli, and salmonella. Prebiotics are foods or nutrients that are used by specific good bacteria, that can be added to the diet to increase the chances of these particular bacteria growing and thriving in the intestine.

It is advisable to take probiotics:
- when suffering from stomach upset, food poisoning, and chronic intestinal problems such as diarrhoea, colitis, constipation and other digestive problems
- after taking antibiotics
- when travelling or vacationing in foreign countries
- when suffering from the fungal infection known as Candida, because probiotics establish large, healthy populations of friendly bacteria that compete with the candida that is trying to take up residence.
- when treating thrush, vaginal yeast infections, and athlete's foot.
- when having dull skin colour and lack of skin elasticity due to intestinal dysfunction
- when suffering from cystitis
- to regulate immune response

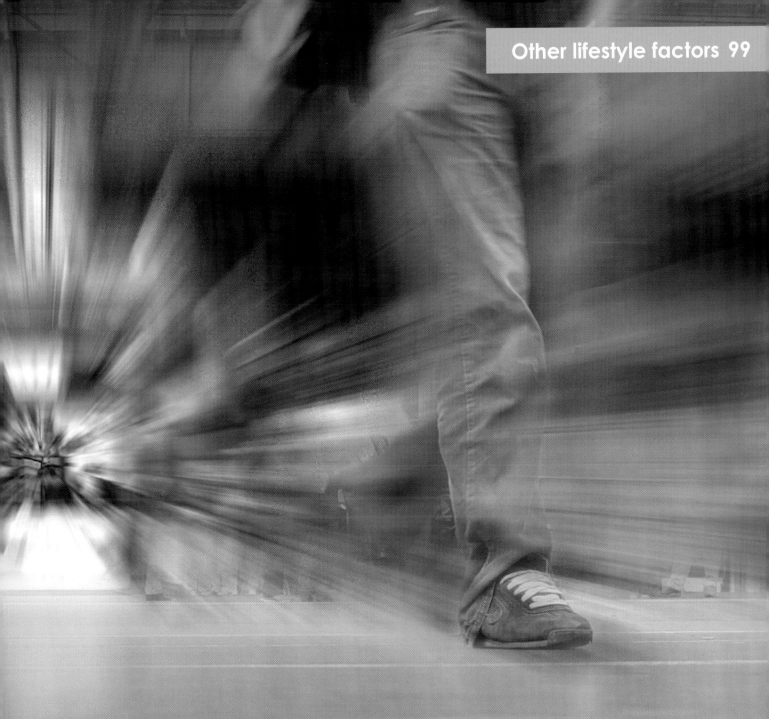

Chapter 7
Other lifestyle
factors

Stress
Immune function
Make up
Hairstyle
Wardrobe

Stress

Stress has been called the silent killer. It weakens your immune system and accelerates ageing. We often race through life with a constantly aroused sympathetic ('fight or flight') nervous system. The adrenal glands, which are a pair of triangle-shaped organs that rest on top of the kidneys, pump out the stress hormones adrenaline and cortisol (an 'ageing' hormone) to help the body cope better with stressful events. It's important to remember that the body reacts to physical, mental, chemical, nutritional, emotional, electromagnetic and microbial stress in the same way – with the excessive release of these hormones, which increase the metabolism. This is known as the alarm stage, and can be a good thing if we need to rise to a challenge.

Problems develop when we function continually in this alarm stage without allowing the body to adequately rest. We feel tired a lot of the time and are aware that we don't have as much energy as we used to. Often we'll rely on stimulants such as strong coffee to keep going, and high blood pressure can result.

Because cortisol suppresses the sleep hormone melatonin, we don't sleep so well, which may result in dark circles under the eyes. This is the resistance stage, and is so called because the body has adapted to this heightened state. This can go on for months or years.

Finally we reach a stage where we look haggard, need medications to sleep and perk us up, and we can barely get out of bed. This is the exhaustion stage or 'burnout'. Our adrenal glands have become exhausted because they cannot keep up with the demand. This is serious because internal organs, including the heart and major blood vessels may be damaged by the effects of prolonged release of adrenalin and cortisol. The wearing out of the adrenal glands frequently leads to an impairment in the thyroid gland, which can cause a further decline in energy level and mood.

Our bodies were designed for short-term stress responses. The longer the stress response, the greater the risk to our health. Long-term release of cortisol also kills memory-forming neurons. And to add insult to injury, the stress response causes the adrenals to decrease production of DHEA. As already discussed, DHEA is a broad-acting hormone that only demonstrates itself under a specific set of circumstances. In that way, it is like a buffer against sudden changes in acidity or alkalinity. That is why when you get older you're much more vulnerable to the effects of stress. As DHEA declines with age, you are losing the buffer against the stress-related hormones.

A further breakthrough was made in 2004 when scientists identified the first direct link between stress and ageing, a finding that goes a long way to explain why intense, long-term emotional strain can make people get sick and grow old before their time.

One study showed that chronic stress appears to hasten the shrivelling of the tips of the bundles of genes inside cells called telomeres, which shortens their life span and speeds the body's deterioration. This is the first time that psychological stress has been linked to a cellular indicator of ageing in healthy people. The study demonstrated that there is no such thing as a separation of mind and body – the very molecules in our bodies are responsive to our psychological environment.[1]

Every time a cell divides, telomeres get shorter. In the natural ageing process, the telomeres eventually get so short that cells can no longer divide, and they then die. As more and more cells reach the end of their telomeres and die, the inexorable process produces the effects of ageing – muscles weaken, skin wrinkles, eyesight and hearing fade, organs fail, and thinking abilities diminish. It is unclear exactly how stress might affect telomeres and telomerase levels, but it could be that chronically elevated levels of stress hormones, such as cortisol, damage the telomeres and other genes in the body and lower telomerase levels, inhibiting the cells' ability to respond.

The team studied 39 women aged 20–50 years who had been experiencing grinding stress for years because they were caring for a child suffering from a serious chronic illness, such as autism or cerebral palsy, and 19 other very similar women whose children were healthy. The researchers examined the telomeres inside cells. The researchers also measured levels of the enzyme telomerase, which helps rebuild telomeres to stave off this process. Telomerase levels naturally decline with age.

The researchers found that chronic stress appears to accelerate this process. The longer a woman had been caring for a sick child, the shorter her telomeres, the lower her levels of telomerase and the higher her levels of oxidative stress (free radical damage to DNA, including telomeres).

This study goes a long way to proving the common perception that unrelenting emotional pressure accelerates the ageing process.

Lower your stress

Stimulants damage the adrenal glands by increasing their activity. Of these there are many. Caffeine, sugar and alcohol are among the most common. Less obvious stimulants include anger, rage, arguing, loud music, suspense and horror movies, and watching the news (especially in the age we are living in). Vigorous exercise also acts as a stimulant, and other stressors in busy cities are noise and electromagnetic pollution from mobile phones and mobile phone masts; televisions, microwave ovens and computers.

Highly strung, nervous individuals and those with very active minds are especially prone to adrenal burnout. Unhealthy responses to stress are an important cause. These include habits of worrying, or becoming angry or afraid.

Sleep is also important for lowering stress. During sleep your adrenal glands are restored and repaired. Unfortunately, most of us get less than we need, night after night, resulting in our adrenal glands staying depleted. The average person needs 6–8 hours of sleep each night. Keys to better sleep include the following:

- Avoid bed-time snacks, particularly refined grains and sugars. These raise blood sugar and inhibit sleep. Later, when blood sugar drops too low (hypoglycemia), you might wake up and not be able to fall back asleep.
- Sleep in complete darkness or as close as possible. When light hits the eyes, it disrupts the circadian rhythm of the pineal gland and production of melatonin and seratonin. There also should be as little light in the bathroom as possible if you get up in the middle of the night.
- No television right before bed, and no TV in the bedroom. It is too stimulating to the brain and you will take longer to fall asleep. Also the pineal gland will not function well for the same reason as above.
- Don't read anything stimulating, such as a mystery or suspense novel just before bed.
- Wear socks to bed. Due to the fact that they have the poorest circulation, the feet often feel cold before the rest of the body, and can wake you up.
- Avoid using loud alarm clocks. It is very stressful on the body to be awoken suddenly. If you are regularly getting enough sleep, they should be unnecessary.

Emotional stress

As mentioned earlier, emotional stress has the same effect on the body as physical and other forms of stress. It's often worse because it affects our very being and peace of mind. If not addressed, it can lead to depression. Here is something to remember.

Believe that all will be well. Sometimes I wish that, when we are going through a turbulent time, we could see the end from the beginning. If we could we would know that above all we're going to be alright. Things will settle down again, and we shall be the stronger, wiser and happier for it. There's been some pain along the way, but it's forgotten because things have resolved themselves – there's a need to put the past behind us and look forward to the future together. To achieve this, I believe that there are two things that we need to know:

The first is that we need to know that joy is not the same as happiness. Happiness comes from humans through fellowship and relationships. People can make us happy, and they can also make us sad. We cannot control it. Joy, on the other hand is where we do have control. Joy is a spiritual force that will get us through any trouble or trial. It is steady and abiding. Our joy is our strength, and with it we can get through anything. Joy comes from a good conscience and a connection with a greater power.

The second, connected to the comments above, is that this whole section has shown just how detrimental to our health stress can be. Simply put, the human body was not designed to deal with stress. I believe that this wasn't a design fault but was deliberate. Unlike other stressors, such as physical, chemical or electromagnetic, where we can rectify the situation by removing ourselves from the stressor (by taking days off work, removing chemicals from our lifestyles etc.), emotional stress is not something that can just go away. We need to give it away. When we do, we find ourselves lighter because we are no longer carrying the burdens. We have found a help that we can rely on.

Immune function

Your body's best defence

As the human body enters its senior years, its ability to fight off infection and other health problems diminishes significantly. The immune system, which is responsible for fighting infection, simply does not function as efficiently in older adults as it does in younger people.

The tell-tale signs that the immune system is weakening include fatigue and lethargy, repeated infections such as colds and flu, slow wound healing and allergies. A healthy adult should suffer no more than two colds a year – so if you do seem to succumb to every passing infection, you definitely need to start supporting your immune system.

The body's innate response to infection – developing a fever to kill cells causing illness, for example – is not always automatic in elderly people. In fact, more than 20% of adults over the age of 65, who have serious bacterial infections, do not have fevers. The body at this age probably still has the ability to generate fevers and other immunity weapons, but the central nervous system is simply less sensitive to immune signals and doesn't react as quickly or efficiently to infection.

Having a strong immune system can help strengthen your body against ageing. Although it is important to note that ageing is not a combination of degenerative and infective disease, but an accumulation of natural processes, staying disease free will not keep you youthful – but it will keep you in good health and better equipped to make the lifestyle changes necessary to beat the ageing process.

Your immune system army

Our immune system can be thought of as your body's armed forces, and each component part has it's specific job to defend the body. It has foot soldiers…

White blood cells

Your immune system's foot soldiers are the body's white blood cells. These cells patrol the bloodstream, preventing microbes from gaining a foothold. There are millions of these microscopic fighters in each drop of blood.

Continuing the army analogy, the special forces would be the macrophages, which are specialised white blood cells that support the other white blood cells in combating invaders.

Further back-up is provided by T-lymphocytes, which are white blood cells originating in the thymus (a tiny gland in front of the heart). The thymus begins to atrophy after adolescence. By middle age it is only about 15% of its maximum size.

Some of the T cells directly kill foreign particles. Others help coordinate other parts of the immune system, which are specialised to attack different types of infections. Although the number of T cells does not decrease with ageing, T cell function decreases. This causes a weakening of the parts of the immune system controlled by these T cells.

Lymphocytes

Lymphocytes, cells produced in the lymph glands, are essential to the body's production of antibodies used to fight infection. The overall number of lymphocytes does not change greatly in old age, but the configuration of lymphocytes and their reaction to infection does.

Elderly adults are less capable of producing lymphocytes to combat challenges to the immune system. The infection-fighting cells that are produced are less vigorous and less effective than those found in younger adults. When antibodies are produced, the duration of their response is shorter in older adults and fewer cells are produced than in younger adults. The immune system of younger adults – including lymphocytes and other types of cells – typically reacts more strongly and more rapidly to infection than does an older adult's.

In addition, elderly adults, particularly after age of 70, are more likely to produce auto-antibodies which cause autoimmune reactions; these attack parts of the body itself instead of infections. Autoimmune responses can cause rheumatoid arthritis and atherosclerosis (hardening of the arteries).

Improving the immune system response

Certain prostaglandins, hormone-like acids that affect important body processes such as body temperature and metabolism, may increase in old age and inhibit important immune cells from doing their jobs. Older adults may also be more sensitive to the action of prostaglandins than younger adults, which could be a major cause of immune deficiency in elderly people. Prostaglandins are produced by most tissues in the body, but the immune system responds better in older adults when prostaglandin production is suppressed.

Older adults often experience loss and stress, and suppressed immunity has been associated with bereavement, depression and poor social support. Maintaining an active social life and receiving treatment for depression could boost the older adult's immune system.

Nutrition plays a factor in a healthy immune system. In both healthy and nutritionally deficient older adults, vitamin and dietary supplements have been found to enhance the response of the immune system, resulting in fewer days of infectious illnesses. It has not been proven that a less effective immune system necessarily means more infections or a shorter life. However, in general, older adults experience more infections and a greater severity of infections than younger adults.

Immune system weakeners

If there's a cold going round, indulge in any of the below and you'll be sure to catch it.

- Consuming refined sugar. Eating or drinking 100 g (8 tbsp) of sugar, the equivalent of about two cans of soda, can reduce the ability of white blood cell to kill germs by 40%. The immune-suppressing effect of sugar starts less than 30 minutes after ingestion and may last for 5 hours. In contrast, the ingestion of complex carbohydrates, or starches, has no effect on the immune system.

- Excess alcohol. Excessive alcohol intake can harm the body's immune system in two ways. First, it produces an overall nutritional deficiency, depriving the body of valuable immune- boosting nutrients. Second, alcohol, like sugar, consumed in excess can reduce the ability of white cells to kill germs. High doses of alcohol suppress the ability of the white blood cells to multiply, inhibit the action of killer white cells on cancer cells, and lessen the ability of macrophages to produce tumour necrosis factors. One drink (the equivalent of 1/2 pint of beer, 175 ml of wine, or 25 ml of spirits) does not appear to bother the immune system, but three or more drinks do. Damage to the immune system increases in proportion to the quantity of alcohol consumed. Amounts of alcohol that are enough to cause intoxication are also enough to suppress immunity.

- Smoking. This will age you: Cut back or, better yet, cut it out altogether.

● Food allergens. Owing to a genetic quirk, some divisions of the immune army recognise an otherwise harmless substance (such as milk) as a foreign invader and attack it, causing an allergic reaction. Before the battle, the intestinal lining was like a wall impenetrable to foreign invaders. After many encounters with food allergens, the wall is damaged, enabling invaders and other potentially toxic substances in the food to get into the bloodstream and make the body feel miserable. This condition is known as the leaky gut syndrome.

● Too much fat. Obesity can lead to a depressed immune system. It can affect the ability of white blood cells to multiply, produce antibodies, and rush to the site of an infection.

Other factors that can help you look younger

● *A pearly white smile.* Whiter teeth are very youthful and will make you look young and youthful. Teeth become discoloured as we age, so the whiter your teeth, the younger you appear. Buy over-the-counter tooth whiteners, which have become very popular, or see your dentist for professional whitening options (see Resources section).

● *Revamp your wardrobe.* Wearing clothes that make you appear youthful doesn't mean mutton dressed as lamb. Many department stores now have stylists who can advise you on changing your look.
Wear the right colours. Wear colours that complement your skin tone and eye colour. See a colour expert (see Resources section).

● *Update your hairstyle or colour.* You wouldn't wear the same outfit for 10 years, so why keep the same hairstyle? Avoid severe blunt cut styles which can be ageing, instead try layered styles which can give you a softer look. If you take your hair one shade lighter, this can brighten and lift your skin tone. Speak to a hairstylist, and don't do anything drastic until you're sure the new look will suit you.

● *Revamp your make-up.* The correct make-up cleverly applied can take years off your looks. Light reflecting make-up can brighten the complexion, and diffuse fine lines and wrinkles. Use a liquid base instead of a powder because powder can settle into fine lines, making you look older. A brightener or concealer around your eyes can hide circles and dark shadows and wake up the eyes, but steer clear of heavy concealers. Brown lipstick can also age you by making your lips appear thinner. Lighter, brighter colours are more youthful. Also, avoid matte lipstick as it tends to settle into any lip lines you may have.

RECIPES

Breakfast

Power Porridge
Serves 1
40 g (1 ½ oz) porridge oats
250 ml (8 fl oz) organic non-homogenised
milk (full fat is allowed) or goat's
milk or almond milk
To sweeten: 5 ml (1 tsp) honey or a few
sultanas/raisins, or ½ mashed banana or 3
chopped organic dates or 3 chopped dried
organic apricots
For added protein add either: 25 g (1 tbsp)
sunflower seeds soaked overnight and
drained or 20 g ground almonds or 20 g
ground hazelnuts or 20 g ground Brazil nuts

1. Mix ingredients together and simmer for
   5–10 minutes.
2. Sweeten with either the honey or fruit.
3. If you want some added protein, add the
   final ingredients and mix thoroughly.

Fruit Smoothie
Serves 2
1 banana
1/3 pineapple
25 g (1 oz) sunflower seeds (soaked overnight
and drained)
120 ml (4 fl oz) fresh fruit juice
Ice

1. Blend all ingredients together.
2. Add ice when needed.

Very Berry Smoothie
Serves 4
10 organic strawberries
2 bananas
250 ml (8 fl oz) fruit juice or milk (see above)
25 g (1 oz) of blueberries
1 kiwi fruit
10 pitted cherries
Ice

1. Blend all ingredients until smooth. Serves 4

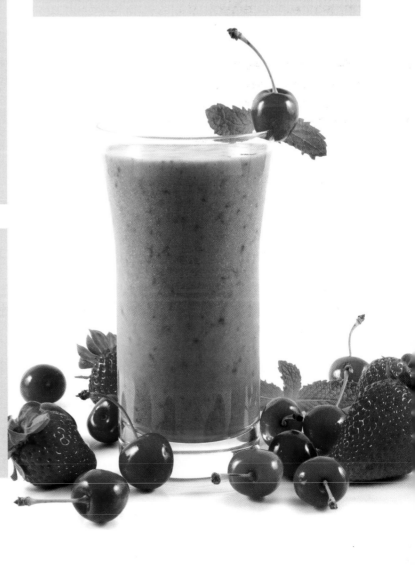

Millet Porridge

Millet is one of the few alkali-forming grains and is especially good for hair. Follow the Power Porridge recipe, replacing the oats with millet flakes (available from health food stores)

Quinoa Porridge

Quinoa is another alkali-forming grain, which contains protein of a better quality than meat, as well as vitamins, minerals, and essential fatty acids. However, unless you're from Peru, where it's a staple part of their diet, I find that the best way to have quinoa is in a porridge. You can get quinoa flakes (from your health food store), and you can use these to make a porridge by replacing half of the porridge oats (recipe above) with the flaked quinoa. Or you can replace half of your oats with 25 g (1 tbsp) of the quinoa grains and simmer in a little water for around 15 minutes until soft (don't let the water dry out), then add to the oats and milk and simmer for a further 10 minutes until creamy.

Eggs

An egg a day or seven per week is allowed on this plan because eggs are an integral part of any anti-ageing plan. Buy only free-range eggs or check that the hens have been able to pasture. This way you are ensuring a plentiful supply of vitamins A and D, omega-3 fats and, of course, protein.
Have them poached, boiled, scrambled or made into an omelette.

Grand Granola
Serves 4

25 g (1 tbsp) sesame seeds
25 g (1 tbsp) sunflower seeds
25 g (1 tbsp) pumpkin seeds
25 g (1 tbsp) shredded coconut
225 g (8 oz) porridge oats
25 g (1 tbsp) chopped almonds
25 g (1 tbsp) chopped pecans
30 ml (2 tbsp) runny honey
70 g (2 ½ oz) raisins

1. Grind together all the seeds and coconut.
2. Mix with remaining ingredients.
3. Spread thinly on a baking sheet
4. Bake at 150ºC (Gas Mark 2) for 20 minutes or until lightly toasted.
5. Leave to cool and store in an airtight container.
6. Serve with organic dairy or rice milk.

Fruity Sundae
Serves 1–2

1 ripe banana
15 ml (1 tbsp) cottage cheese
6 grapes, halved
5 g (1 tsp) wheat germ
2 g (½ tsp) cinnamon
6 sliced strawberries
30–45 ml (2–3 tbsp) natural yoghurt
5 ml (1 tsp) honey
25 g (1 tbsp) chopped pecans

1. Cut banana length-wise and place in a bowl.
2. Combine cheese with grapes, wheat germ, and cinnamon.
3. Form into a scoop and set in middle of banana.
4. Top with strawberries and yoghurt and honey.
5. Sprinkle with nuts.

Healthy English Breakfast
Serves 1
Egg
2 turkey rashers or 2 slices of lean organic bacon
25 g (1 tbsp) baked beans (no sugar and salt, try organic)
Small handful of mushrooms
2 tomatoes

1. Poach or boil the egg.
2. Grill the turkey rashers.
3. Grill mushrooms and tomatoes
4. Serve with pitta bread or a slice of who legrain toast.

Fruit & Cereal
Serves 2
1 apple
1 peach
25 g (1 tbsp) blueberries
1 banana
6 grapes
25 g (1 tbsp) granola
15 ml (1 tbsp) yoghurt
10 ml (2 tsp) honey

1. Wash and core fruit leaving on peel.
2. Dice and place half in each bowl.
3. Sprinkle with granola.
4. Top with yoghurt and sweeten with honey.

Lunch and dinner recipes

If these recipes are not for you, devise your own, using the food tables on pages 23-27, making sure that you focus on the foods and guidelines listed in the table.

Vegetables and vegetarian recipes

Tomatoes are an important part of the anti-ageing diet. They contain lycopene, which can protect the skin against UV damage. Try to eat tomato-based stews, casseroles and stir-fries at least three times per week. With this base you can prepare a multitude of dishes.

Tomato Base
45 ml (3 tbsp) extra virgin olive oil
10 ml (2 tsp) virgin coconut oil
1 onion, sliced
1 clove garlic, chopped (optional)
Small pinch chilli powder
(according to taste)
1 x 400 g tin of plum tomatoes
30 ml (2 tbsp) tomato purée
Pinch of dried parsley
1 organic vegetable stock cube
(organic contains no MSG)

1. Heat oils together and add sliced onions; fry for 5 minutes.
2. Add garlic. (At this stage, you can add a chicken breast, diced lamb or other meat).
3. Add the chilli, tomatoes, stock cube, tomato purée and parsley and bring to the boil; simmer on low heat for 15–20 minutes.

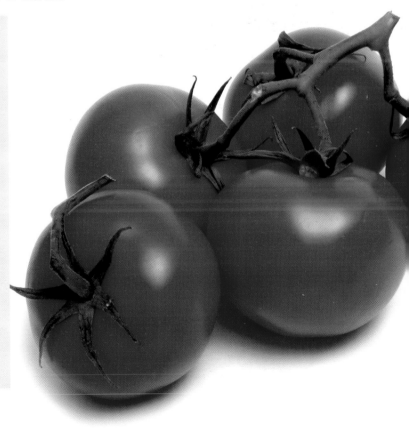

Greens and Tomatoes

This recipe uses all the ingredients in the Tomato Base recipe with the addition of 900 g (2 lb) greens, washed thoroughly. Cut any tough stems out of leaves, and cut or tear the leaves into bite-size pieces.

Serves 4

1. Rinse torn leaves well; but do not dry.
2. Put wet leaves in a large pan with a sprinkle of sea salt and let wilt over medium–low heat, stirring constantly. Now follow the steps in the tomato base recipe above.
3. After adding the chilli, tomatoes, purée and stock cube, bring to the boil, then add the prepared greens. Simmer covered for 15 minutes.
4. Serve with basmati rice.

Spinach and Red Peppers

Serves 2

15 ml (1 tbsp) extra virgin olive oil
8 g (1/4 tsp) butter
10 ml (2 tsp) virgin coconut oil
2 medium red peppers, deseeded and cut into strips
2 garlic cloves, very thinly sliced
1 pinch crushed red pepper flakes
600 g (1 ½ lb) fresh rinsed spinach
Pinch sea salt, or to taste

1. In a large frying pan, heat the butter, coconut and olive oil over a medium heat.
2. Add the peppers, garlic, and pepper flakes. Cook, stirring frequently, for about 4 minutes.
3. Add the (undried) spinach to the pan. Sprinkle with salt. Increase heat to medium–high and cook, stirring occasionally, for 3 minutes or until vegetables are tender.

Greens and Parmesan Casserole

Serves 4

650 g (1 ½ lb) greens, washed and trimmed (try kale for a change), cutting out the tough ribs if necessary
Salt and freshly ground black pepper
1 cup chicken or vegetable broth
60 g (2 ¼ oz) butter
60 ml (2 tbsp) virgin coconut oil
25 g (1 tbsp) flour
25 g (1 tbsp) grated Parmesan cheese
50 g (2 tbsp) ricotta cheese (whole milk or semi-skimmed)
75 g (3 tbsp) dry bread crumbs
50 g (2 tbsp) Mozzarella cheese, shredded

1. Butter baking or casserole dish; preheat the oven to 150°C (Gas Mark 2).
2. Chop the prepared greens into 12.5 mm (½ in) pieces.
3. In a large frying pan, cook the greens over low heat, adding them by handfuls and stirring them down as they wilt. Add 1/2 cup of water if the greens seem dry, then cover the pan and braise for 10–15 minutes, or until tender. Pour off any liquid left in the pan, then season the greens with salt and pepper. Transfer to a bowl and set aside.
4. Heat the broth in a saucepan, just until bubbles form around the edge of the pan.
5. In the large frying pan, melt the butter and coconut oil over low heat.
6. Add the flour and cook, stirring, for 1 minute.
7. Add the hot broth mixture all at once and stir over medium heat until the sauce is smooth and thickened.
8. Whisk in the grated Parmesan and ricotta.
9. Stir the greens into the cheese sauce and pour the mixture into the prepared casserole dish.
10. Sprinkle over the bread crumbs and finally the grated mozzarella over the top.
11. Bake for 20 minutes, or until the sauce is bubbling and the mozzarella is melted and lightly browned. Serve immediately.

Non-meat proteins

Walnut and Cashew Pesto
Serves 4

100 g (3 1/2 oz) walnut pieces
100 g (3 1/2 oz) cashew nuts
1 bunch of basil
1 bunch spinach
4 cloves of garlic
120 ml (8 tbsp) extra virgin olive oil or Ultimate Oil Blend (see Suppliers list)
Pinch sea salt and freshly ground black pepper

1. Lightly toast the nuts in a medium oven.
2. Pick basil leaves from stems and place in a blender with all the other ingredients.
3. Add the nuts and blend.
4. Chill in the fridge.

Hummus
Serves 4

1 X 400 g tin chick peas
1 clove garlic
15 ml (1 tbsp) extra virgin olive oil or Udos Ultimate Oil Blend
30 ml (2 tbsp) light tahini
Juice of 1/2 lemon
Pinch of cayenne or paprika (optional)

1. Mix all the ingredients together until creamy.
2. Chill in the fridge

Feta Pitta Sandwich
Serves 2

3 pitta breads, cut in half
4 cubes of Feta cheese
1 large ripe tomato, sliced
1 medium carrot, grated
1 cup parsley, chopped
Alfafa sprouts
Leaf lettuce

1. Toast the pitas, then stuff with ingredients.

Falafel Burgers
Serves 3

175 ml (6 fl oz) water (or follow direction on packet)
1 cup falafel mix
15 ml (1 tbsp) olive oil
Pitta bread
Alfalfa sprouts
Tomatoes
Ketchup

1. Add water to falafel mix. Let it stand for 15 minutes or until water is absorbed.
2. Form into patties and fry in oil until brown on each side.
3. Serve in pitta bread with sprouts, tomatoes, and your favourite condiments.

Soups

Chicken Soup
You don't have to be Jewish to enjoy home-made chicken soup. This dish is classic comfort food, and has acquired the reputation as a remedy for colds, 'flu and other illnesses. This may be because of the ingredients, which include plenty of vegetables, calcium and other minerals from the chicken bones. You can double the ingredients and keep the remainder refrigerated, so you have a ready-prepared meal.

Serves 2

1 chicken quarter
1.15 litres (2 pints) water
Freshly ground black pepper
1/2 organic vegetable stock cube
1 large leek
1 onion
1 large carrot

1. Boil the chicken for 1 hour on a very low heat with salt, pepper and the stock cube.
2. Remove the chicken, then add the leek, onion and carrot, and boil for another 15 minutes.
3. The chicken meat can be chopped up and added to the soup if you wish.

Vegetable Soup
Serves 4

25 g (1 oz) butter
10 ml (2 tsp) virgin coconut oil
2 tomatoes, chopped
1 onion, chopped
2 parsley sprigs chopped
50 g (2 oz) shredded cabbage
50g (2 oz) Spinach leaves, chopped
150 g (5 oz) grated carrots
150 g (5 oz) fresh peas
500 ml (17 fl oz) water
Garlic powder and other seasonings of choice

1. Melt butter and oil on low heat and add the vegetables. Cover and let steam for 5 minutes.
2. Add water, heat, then add the garlic and seasonings.

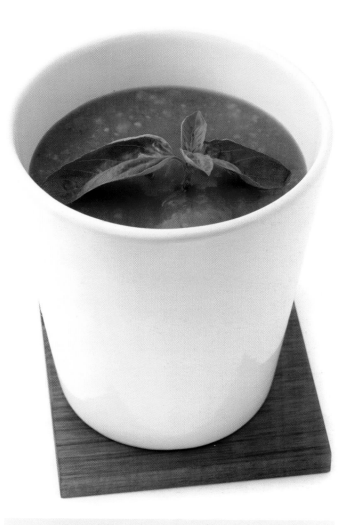

Sweetcorn Soup
Serves 4

1 small onion, chopped
1/2 sweet red pepper, finely chopped
10 ml (2 tsp) olive oil
10 ml (2 tsp) virgin coconut oil
8 g (¼ oz) butter
20 g (2 tsp) whole wheat flour
250 ml (8 fl oz) oat or rice milk
125 ml (4 fl oz) yoghurt
10 ml (2 tsp) tamari soy sauce
250 g (9 oz) fresh sweetcorn
Pinch nutmeg
Parsley, for garnish

1. In a frying pan, cook the onion and pepper in the oils and butter until tender.
2. Stir in flour and soy sauce and heat on low for 2–3 minutes.
3. Add milk slowly.
4. Blend in a food processor the yogurt and two-thirds of the sweetcorn until smooth and add to the creamy mixture with the remaining corn.
5. Heat and serve with nutmeg and parsley.

Tomato Soup
Serves 6

3 cloves garlic, crushed
30 ml (2 tbsp) extra virgin olive oil
10 ml virgin coconut oil
125 g (1 tbsp) paprika
2.25 litres (4 pints) tomato juice or undrained canned tomatoes, puréed in blender 1 organic vegetable stock cube
15 ml (1 tbsp) organic double cream
Croutons
Parmesan cheese, freshly grated
Parsley, freshly chopped

1. Sauté the garlic in oils briefly; do not brown.
2. Stir in paprika and saute for another minute, stirring continuously to avoid scorching.
3. Stir in tomato juice and heat.
4. Add the stock cube and cream. Simmer in a covered pan for 5–10 minutes.
5. Garnish with croutons, cheese and parsley.

Salads

Vegetable Salad

Serves 4

Leaf lettuce
Spinach
Carrots, grated
Green pepper, chopped
Spring onions, chopped
Alfalfa sprouts
Broccoli, chopped
Tomatoes
Parsley
Salad dressing

1. Combine all the ingredients in a large bowl.
2. Serve with dressing.

Garlic Herb Dressing

1 egg
5 ml (1 tsp) Dijon mustard
30 ml (2 tbsp) flax oil or Ultimate Oil blend
1 clove garlic, crushed
15 ml (1 tbsp) lemon juice
25 g (1 oz) fresh parsley
15 ml (1 tbsp) apple cider vinegar
25 g (1 oz) chopped spring onion
25 g (1 oz) fresh basil

1. Place egg and mustard in blender; process on low until beaten well.
2. Add the oil very slowly while blender is still running.
3. Add remaining ingredients, blend well on low and chill.
4. Use on green salads and cooled vegetables.

Meat, Poultry and Fish

Grilled Sardines

Serves 2

500g (1 lb) fresh sardines
45 ml (3 tbsp) olive oil
2 fresh sprigs rosemary
Pinch sea salt
Lemon wedges to garnish

1. Preheat the grill.
2. Leave the heads on the sardines but slit half-way along the belly and clean thoroughly under cold running water. Pat dry with kitchen towel and arrange on the grill pan or baking sheet.
3. Brush sardines with oil and sprinkle with half the fresh rosemary leaves and a little sea salt.
4. Grill for 4–5 minutes until just beginning to brown.
5. Turn the sardines over and brush with more oil and sprinkle with the rest of the rosemary and salt. Grill for a further 4–5 minutes.
6. Serve with sautéed spinach.

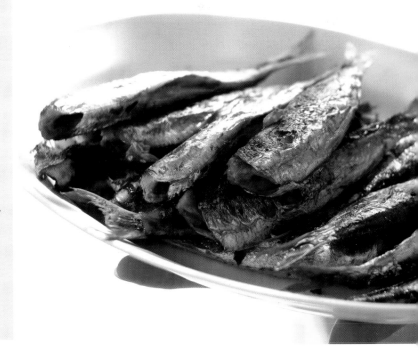

Chicken Casserole

Serves 6
25 g (1 oz) butter
10 ml (2 tsp) virgin coconut oil
15 ml (1 tbsp) extra virgin olive oil
6 chicken drumsticks
5 medium sized organic carrots, chopped
75 g (2 ¾ oz) button mushrooms
1 clove garlic, crushed and minced
1 tsp dried basil
1 tsp ground thyme
25 g (1 oz) flour
15 ml (1 tbsp) organic double cream
200 ml (7 fl oz) chicken broth
Salt and freshly ground black pepper
50 g (2 oz) grated Parmesan cheese

1. In a large pan, melt half the butter and oils; add chicken and brown for 10 minutes.
2. Add carrots, mushrooms, minced garlic, basil, and thyme. Cook over medium–low heat, stirring constantly, for about 5 minutes.
3. Add flour and blend well.
4. Simmer for 5 minutes, stirring constantly.
5. Over medium–low heat, melt remaining butter and blend in remaining flour, stirring until smooth.
6. Gradually stir in double cream and chicken broth; continue cooking and stirring until thickened.
7. Season to taste with salt and pepper. Put everything together in a casserole dish and sprinkle with grated Parmesan cheese.
8. Bake at 150°C (Gas Mark 2) for 50 minutes, until cheese is lightly browned.
9. Serve with basmati rice.

Chicken and Cashew Stir-Fry

Stir-fries make excellent lunches and dinners while you are on this Programme. They're full of vegetables, and are very tasty, so do try to make them a regular meal. You can easily vary the ingredients, just throw in whatever vegetables you fancy. You can also substitute Basmati rice or fragrant Thai rice for the rice noodles. This dish is also delicious cold, so any leftovers are ideal for lunch the next day. Remember to do all your slicing before you start cooking.

Serves 2
1 organic chicken breast fillet
1 egg white
20 g (2 tsp) cornflour
75 g (2 ¾ oz) very thin white rice noodles (e.g. Sharwoods)
45 ml (3 tbsp) olive oil
1 clove of garlic, crushed
1 bunch of spring onions, finely chopped
2 carrots, chopped into thin strips
6 button mushrooms, chopped
50 g (2 oz) frozen peas
50 g (2 oz) sweet peppers (fresh or frozen), very finely chopped
Small knob of fresh ginger, finely chopped
40 g (1 ½ oz) cashew nuts
15 ml (1 tbsp) Bragg's Liquid Aminos (available from health food stores)

1. Slice the chicken into small thin strips.
2. Whisk the egg white with the cornflour; put the chicken in this mixture and refrigerate.
3. Place the noodles in a bowl and cover with boiling water. Cover and leave for 4 minutes, then immediately drain in a sieve.
4. Heat the oil in a wok and add garlic, spring onions and chicken from the fridge (with the mixture included), and stir-fry for 1 minute.
5. Add all the other vegetables plus the ginger and cashew nuts and stir fry for 8–10 minutes or until vegetables have lost their crispness.
6. Add the Liquid Aminos and noodles; mix and serve immediately.

Spaghetti Bolognese

Serves 4

3 carrots

1 onion

50 g (2 oz) sweetcorn

_ a head of broccoli

1 clove garlic

1 x 400 g tin plum tomatoes

400 g (14 oz) organic minced lamb

Pinch cayenne pepper

Pinch Italian herbs

Pinch sea salt

45 ml (3 tbsp) extra virgin Olive oil

10 ml (2 tsp) virgin coconut oil

1. Peel, wash and chop all of the vegetables.
2. Lightly fry the first five vegetables in the oils, then add the tomatoes, mince, cayenne, herbs and sea salt.
3. Leave to simmer for 10 minutes.
4. Serve on cooked wholegrain spaghetti or basmati rice.

Sweets and snacks

Eating well does not mean 'no pudding'. There are plenty of foods that can sweeten just as well as refined sugar. And you can also snack or have a pudding consisting of a handful of goji berries and some mixed nuts.

Oatmeal Cookies

Makes 10 cookies

125g (5 oz) butter

1 tsp vanilla extract

Pinch of sea salt

90 ml (6 tbsp) runny honey

1 tsp lemon rind

175 g (6 oz) organic wholewheat flour or spelt flour

50 ml (1 fl oz) cold water

175 g (6 oz) whole oats

50g (2 oz) almonds, chopped

1. Cream together first 5 ingredients.
2. Mix in the flour and water and add oats and nuts.
3. Mix well and shape into a ball then flatten and place onto a greased baking sheet; flatten with a fork.
4. Bake at 175°C (150°C if using a fan oven) (Gas Mark 2–3) for 15–20 minutes or until brown.

Nut Butter Cookies

Make sure you bake these cookies, and the oatmeal cookies with someone else around, otherwise, because they're so moreish you may end up eating more that you bargained for.

Makes 8 cookies

30 ml (2 tbsp) almond butter or organic peanut butter

15 ml (1 tbsp) extra virgin olive oil

 tsp vanilla extract

30 ml (2 tbsp) honey

100 g (4 oz) organic wholemeal flour or spelt flour

1. Cream all the ingredients together except flour.
2. Slowly stir in flour to make thick dough.
3. Form into 5 cm (2 in) balls, place on baking sheet and flatten with fork.
4. Bake at 175°C (150°C if using a fan oven (Gas Mark 2–3) for 10 minutes.

Chocolate Dipped Strawberries

Use only organic strawberries, and the darkest chocolate you can find which is a good source of antioxidants.

Serves 4

300 g (12 oz) organic strawberries
100 g (4 oz) dark chocolate (70 or
85% cocoa solids – try Green & Blacks)

1. Melt the chocolate in a glass bowl over a saucepan of gently simmering water. Stir until smooth and glossy.
2. Wash the strawberries and pat them dry (any moisture from the fruit will spoil the texture of the melted chocolate).
3. Dip each strawberry into the melted chocolate, covering the lower half of the strawberry. Place on a baking sheet lined with greaseproof paper. Refrigerate for at least 1 hour.

Summer Berry Salad

This delicious, nutritious dish will also make a great breakfast.

Serves 4

150 g (6 oz) organic strawberries
1 large nectarine, sliced
100 g (4 oz) blueberries
2 kiwifruit, peeled
1 large mango
60 ml (4 tbsp) apple juice

1. Combine all the fruit in large bowl.
2. Pour over apple juice.
3. Chill for at least 2 hours.

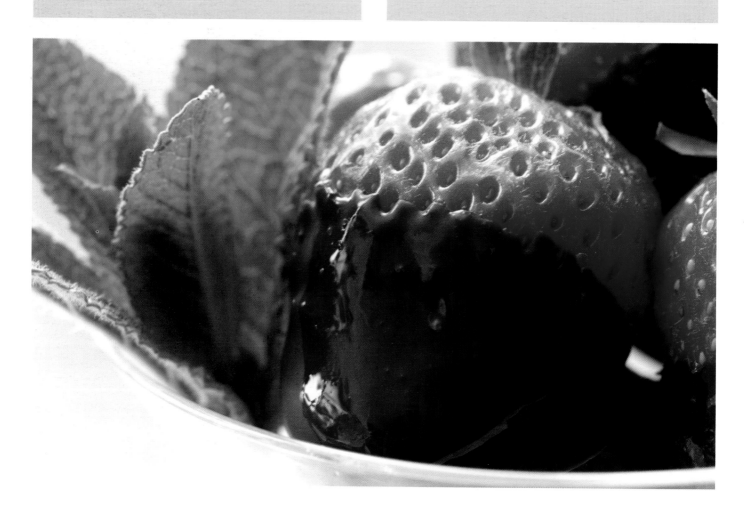

Blueberry Tart

If you're having a dinner party and are looking for a delicious dessert that won't go straight to the hips, try this. I use Smatana in this recipe, which is a low-fat soured cream originally from Russia and Eastern Europe (where it's known as Smetana), and has less fat than traditional soured cream or crème fraîche. It's available in the cream section in most supermarkets. I sometimes double the ingredients and use a 25 cm (10 in) round cake tin for a larger tart.

Serves 12

Base
175 g (78 oz) butter, softened
25 g (1 oz) unrefined sugar
100 g (4 oz) organic self-raising flour
100 g (4 oz) organic wholemeal self-raising flour or spelt flour
2 eggs (free range)

Filling
250 g (10 oz) blueberries
284 ml(½ pint) Smatana
2 eggs (free range)
1 tsp vanilla extract
25 g (1 oz) unrefined sugar

1. Pre-heat oven to 175°C (150°C if using a fan oven) (Gas Mark 2–3).
2. Line a 25 cm (10 in) round cake tine with baking parchment or paper.
3. Cream the butter and sugar with a hand-held electric hand mixer.
4. Add the egg, then the flours.
5. Place the mixture in the tin to form the base of the tart, and place the blueberries on the base.
6. Beat the Smatana, egg, vanilla and sugar together with a hand-held electric mixer then pour over the blueberries.
7. Bake in the oven for around 30 minutes or until it's golden brown and the filling is just set. If it seems too wobbly, don't worry, it will firm as it cools.
8. Allow to cool. It's delicious served both warm and cold, and tastes just as good if baked the day before, refrigerated over night and served at room temperature the next day.

Optional

To really impress, make a blueberry or fruit coulis as an accompaniment (a healthier alternative to clotted cream, though a little clotted cream is allowed only very occasionally and in moderation). Simply simmer fresh blueberries (or other berries, or use a bag of store-bought frozen summer fruits) in a little apple juice, whiz in a processor and strain through a sieve. Serve hot or cold.

Melon Berry Salad

Serves 4
1 cantaloupe melon peeled, sliced and chopped
150 g (6 oz) fresh organic strawberries
150 g (6 oz) fresh raspberries
150g (6 oz) fresh blueberries
1 tbsp honey
45 ml (3 tbsp) apple juice

1. Combine fruit in large bowl.
2. Pour over apple juice.
3. Chill for at least 2 hours.

Your 12-week programme

After 12 weeks on the programme you will observe physiological changes such as increased energy, elevated mood, improved sleep, increased stamina, improved memory, changes in cholesterol and increased libido.

Physical changes include improved muscle tone, decreased body fat, improved skin tone, a reduction in skin wrinkling and improved hair condition. A reminder that this Programme is all about incorporating anti-ageing changes into your lifestyle without any upheaval or inconvenience. It lasts for 12 weeks, not so that you follow it for this amount of time, achieve results, then revert back to old habits. No, it's 12 weeks because it takes this long to see sustainable improvements in your health and appearance, and during this time you have incorporated new behaviours into your lifestyle until they become established habits.

A reminder that the four components are:
- Incorporate rebounding and walking into your physical activity programme
- Modify your diet
- Supplement
- Use anti-ageing skincare

The Rebounder Programme

First things first, you don't want a young face and body and drooping breasts, so make sure you invest in a firm fitting sports bra before you start rebounding. I recommend the Shock Absorber. I'm full busted myself and can attest that when jumping on my trampoline in my Shock Absorber bra, they barely move.

Rebounding is such a good form of exercise because it is so easy to do. You don't need an instructional video, you don't need to go to a class, all you need to do is get onto your Rebounder and jump! It's that simple.

To guide you through, I have devised a 12-week programme. It is important to start gently, just 1 minute or less at a time if you are new to exercise. When you are tired, stop. It is important to listen to you body and to do what it tells you. Remember that the quality of your rebounder is important – a poor quality rebounder will make rebounding unpleasant and you will not want to do it or it may cause injury. I recommend Trimilin rebounders. See the Resources section for where to purchase them.

Keep your Rebounder in sight so that you can jump on it at any time for a quick workout. In addition to the time set aside for your rebounding, try to do 3–5 minutes (the more the better) of rebounding 15–20 minutes before a meal.

Use triggers to get onto the Rebounder, such as every time you hear a news bulletin, or whenever your favourite soap is on.

The best tip when beginning an exercise programme is to try and get it out of the way early. That way you've got your day off to a healthful start, and you feel good.

Always start off with a warm-up, and end your workouts with the stretches featured on pages 65 and 67.

If you are unsure on your feet and feel you may need a support bar, see the Resources section for how to purchase one.

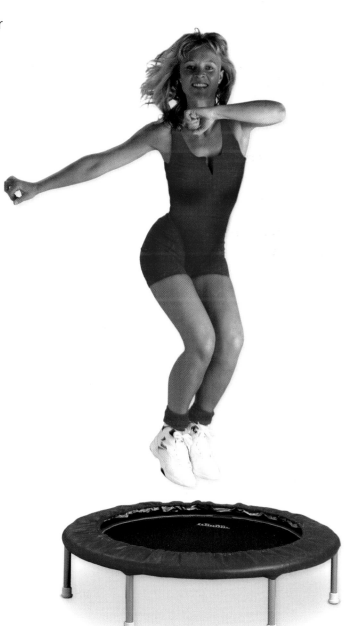

Frequency

Week 1:   5–7 minutes 2 or 3 times per day

Week 2:   10 minutes 1 or 2 times per day

Week 3:   15 minutes 1 or 2 times per day

Week 4:   20 minutes 1 or 2 times per day

Week 5:   20 minutes once a day

Week 6:   20 minutes once a day

Week 7:   25 minutes once a day

Week 8:   25 minutes once a day

Week 9:   25 minutes once a day

Week 10: 30 minutes once a day

Week 11: 30 minutes once a day

Week 12: 30 minutes once a day

The bounces

The warm-up bounce

Bounce lightly up and down lifting heels but keeping the soles of your feet on the mat.

The CV bounce

Slowly jog on the Rebounder.

The High bounce

Jump up and down with both feet landing at the same time. The higher the bounce, the stronger the G-force felt.

High jumps

Jump as high as possible tucking legs under bottom and using arms for balance, or reaching arms forward and down, bringing feet above your hands (both very advanced and only for the very fit).

Skipping

Skip as you would on the ground at your own pace (only for the very fit).

Workouts

Put on your favourite music (up-tempo). Always start with a 1–2 minute warm-up consisting of the Warm-up and CV bounces, then progress to a combination of all bounces.

Always cool down by doing more Warm-up and CV bounces, then do the stretches.

From week 4 (or, if you are already used to exercise, from week 1), add the toning exercises on page 57-63 to your work-out, after the cool-down and before the stretches.

Just bounce

When you don't feel like doing a workout, just get on to the rebounder and bounce. It will make a difference.

Points to remember whilst rebounding

- The Rebounder mat can be a little slippery when cold, so be careful as you are warming up.
- Do not rebound in your socks – have bare-feet or trainers (trainers recommended).
- Perform all exercises using the correct technique and in a controlled manner. If any exercise causes discomfort or pain, stop immediately.
- Maintain rhythmical breathing whilst rebounding. You should be able to hold a conversation during the main component of your workout.
- Avoid holding your breath!
- Wear comfortable clothing.
- Ensure you drink plenty of water, before, during and after your workout.
- Always ensure that the 'legs' on your Rebounder are screwed in tightly and that there are no springs missing.
- Stand with your feet hip width apart whilst on the Rebounder and maintain a neutral S-shaped spine whilst exercising.
- Always pull in your abdominal muscles while performing exercises on the Rebounder, as this helps you to stabilise and balance.
- Always try to maintain a central position on the rebounder and avoid bouncing onto the floor!

Some helpful hints

- Take the phone off the hook or turn the ringer off so that you are not disturbed.
- Ensure you have a clear area in which to put your rebounder, checking for any low-hanging ceiling lights.
- Apart from the suggested workouts per week, if you have a spare moment, jump onto your Rebounder.

The Eating Plan

Top tips

- Avoid sugar (healthy skin's worst enemy).
- Avoid polyunsaturated fats (unless they are cold-pressed), hydrogenated and trans fats. Use extra virgin olive oil, coconut oil, butter and use a cold-pressed omega 3 and 6 oil such as Udo's oil.
- Have a cooked tomato dish 3 days per week.
- Have a green leafy vegetables dish 3 days per week.
- Base your meals around the foods contained in the table of anti-ageing foods on page 23-27.
- Have a handful of goji berries daily.
- A water ioniser is a wise anti-ageing investment (see the Resources section). Drink ionised water frequently every day and use the acid water for cleaning skin.

Also, try to:

- Eat food as close to its natural state as possible.
- Eat some fresh, raw produce with every meal (such as a small side salad or fruit beforehand).
- Avoid coffee, and excessive alcohol consumption as they are all acid-forming and dehydrating.
- Avoid too much salt (use sea salt moderately) and salty foods.

And in addition:

- Don't buy fruit, vegetables, or ice-cream from the road-side where they have been exposed to exhaust fumes.
- Don't cook in aluminium or non-stick pans, use stainless steel or cast iron.
- Steer clear of tobacco smoke and exhaust fumes.
- Restrict the use of the microwave, and only use with glass or ceramic containers, never plastic.

Remember:

- Don't rely on willpower alone, change the way you think about food, see it as the means to youthful health and vitality.
- Change your eating habits slowly, don't attempt it overnight
- Good nutrition is as much about what you don't eat as what you eat.
- Aim for three good meals daily, and healthy snacks in between these meals.

Your 12-week progress diary

Keeping a progress diary is a useful tool to chart progress and encourage you to keep going. Keeping a diary shows you what you're doing each day, and enables you to identify your weak spots and improve them; it also gives you an opportunity to think about yourself and write down your thoughts.

Try to complete it daily – often you won't get round to catching up if you miss a few days. It will help keep you disciplined and on track. Don't by any means be despondent if you miss a day or two of rebounding or walking. Just pick up where you left off and you'll soon be back on track.

Vital measures

When starting off, measure your height and weight to determine your BMI (body mass index). Also measure your waist size and if you have access, get your percentage body fat measured by someone who measures skin-fold thicknesses using Harpenden Callipers. You could try your GP or a local health club. Assess the results using the tables as shown.

Try not to weigh yourself too much whilst on the Programme. This is not about weight loss, it's about developing muscle to tone the body and increase your metabolism, losing excess fat, improving skin tone and other beneficial changes to make you look and feel younger. As well as using the BMI, waist size and percentage body fat tables, use these indicators as your measure for progress:

- How much stronger and fitter do you feel?
- Does your body look more toned?
- Does your skin feel firmer and is your complexion clearer?
- Has your hair condition improved?

BMI chart

BMI (kg/m²)	19	20	21	22	23	24	25	26	27	28	29	30	35	40
Height (in)	Weight (lb)													
58	91	96	100	105	110	115	119	124	129	134	138	143	167	191
59	94	99	104	109	114	119	124	128	133	138	143	148	173	198
60	97	102	107	112	118	123	128	133	138	143	148	153	179	204
61	100	106	111	116	122	127	132	137	143	148	153	158	185	211
62	104	109	115	120	126	131	136	142	147	153	158	164	191	218
63	107	113	118	124	130	135	141	146	152	158	163	169	197	225
64	110	116	122	128	134	140	145	151	157	163	169	174	204	232
65	114	120	126	132	138	144	150	156	162	168	174	180	210	240
66	118	124	130	136	142	148	155	161	167	173	179	186	216	247
67	121	127	134	140	146	153	159	166	172	178	185	191	223	255
68	125	131	138	144	151	158	164	171	177	184	190	197	230	262
69	128	135	142	149	155	162	169	176	182	189	196	203	236	270
70	132	139	146	153	160	167	174	181	188	195	202	207	243	278
71	136	143	150	157	165	172	179	186	193	200	208	215	250	286
72	140	147	154	162	169	177	184	191	199	206	213	221	258	294
73	144	151	159	166	174	182	189	197	204	212	219	227	265	302
74	148	155	163	171	179	186	194	202	210	218	225	233	272	311
75	152	160	168	176	184	192	200	208	216	224	232	240	279	319
76	156	164	172	180	189	197	205	213	221	230	238	246	287	328

BMI	
18.5 or less	Underweight
18.5–24.9	Normal
25.0–29.9	Overweight
30.0–34.9	Obese
35.0–39.9	Obese
40 or more	Extremely obese

Waist size

If your waist measurement is 81 cm (32 in) you're at a higher risk of health problems. Having a waist measurement of over 88 cm (35 in) indicates the highest risk of cardiovascular and metabolic disease. The measurements for men are over 94 cm (37 in) to be at risk of health problems, and 102 cm (40 in) to be at the highest risk for cardiovascular and metabolic diseases.

Percentage body fat

Age	Athlete (%)	Lean (%)	OK (%)	Not Good (%)
19–24	18.9	22.1	25.0	29.6
25–29	18.9	22.0	25.4	29.8
30–34	19.7	22.7	26.4	30.5
35–39	21.0	24.0	27.7	31.5
40–44	22.6	25.6	29.3	32.8
45–49	24.3	27.3	30.9	34.1
50–54	26.6	29.7	33.1	36.2
55–59	27.4	30.7	34.0	37.3
60+	27.6	31.0	34.4	38.0

Your daily routine

On the following pages try to tick off each box daily as you achieve each of the following items.

Exercise

Rebounding on a trampoline 5 days per week (see page 119 for rebounding programme).

Also try to walk 10,000 steps at least 3–4 days per week (I recommend MBTs for this).

Eating plan

A reminder to:

- Avoid sugar.
- Avoid refined carbohydrates such as white bread, cakes, pastries, biscuits and other white flour products and processed foods.
- Avoid polyunsaturated fats (unless they are cold-pressed), hydrogenated and trans fats.
- Use extra virgin olive oil, coconut oil, butter and use a cold-pressed omega 3 and 6 oil such as Udo's oil.
- Have a cooked tomato dish 3 days per week.
- Have a green leafy vegetables dish 3 days per week.
- Base your meals around the foods contained in the table of anti-ageing foods on page 23-27.
- Have a handful of goji berries daily.
- Drink 1½ –2 litres of ionised water every day.

Supplements

- Take Protective Nutrients.
- Take Anti-Ageing Skin, Hair, Nails Formula.

Skin care

- Try to use oil-based skincare, especially moisturisers (see the Resources section).

Measurement	Week 1	Week 12
Waist size		
Percentage body fat		
Weight		

Week One

'Once begun, a task is easy; half the work is done'
Horace

Helpful hints: The best strategy for success on the plan is to get things over with early, that way you've got it out of the way, and can then concentrate on the day feeling good that you've got your body off to a great start. If you leave it till the end of the day, there is a good chance that you won't do it.

Eat fruit early in the day as well. Have a couple of pieces with your breakfast, and as your mid-morning snack. That way, you have got off to a healthful start and are more likely to continue to eat healthily throughout the day.

DAY		NOTES
MONDAY ☐ Exercise ☐ Eating Plan ☐ Supplement ☐ Skincare	● 2-3 x 5-7 min rebounding ● Walked 10,000 steps ● Had greens & tomato-based dish ● Drank 1.5 litres water ● Protective Nutrients Formula ● Skin, Hair, Nails Formula ● Used plant-oil based products	eg: Feeling a lot stronger. Skin looks firm and clear. Trousers seem looser
TUESDAY ☐ Exercise ☐ Eating Plan ☐ Supplement ☐ Skincare	● 2-3 x 5-7 min rebounding ● Walked 10,000 steps ● Had greens & tomato-based dish ● Drank 1.5 litres water ● Protective Nutrients Formula ● Skin, Hair, Nails Formula ● Used plant-oil based products	
WEDNESDAY ☐ Exercise ☐ Eating Plan ☐ Supplement ☐ Skincare	● 2-3 x 5-7 min rebounding ● Walked 10,000 steps ● Had greens & tomato-based dish ● Drank 1.5 litres water ● Protective Nutrients Formula ● Skin, Hair, Nails Formula ● Used plant-oil based products	
THURSDAY ☐ Exercise ☐ Eating Plan ☐ Supplement ☐ Skincare	● 2-3 x 5-7 min rebounding ● Walked 10,000 steps ● Had greens & tomato-based dish ● Drank 1.5 litres water ● Protective Nutrients Formula ● Skin, Hair, Nails Formula ● Used plant-oil based products	
FRIDAY ☐ Exercise ☐ Eating Plan ☐ Supplement ☐ Skincare	● 2-3 x 5-7 min rebounding ● Walked 10,000 steps ● Had greens & tomato-based dish ● Drank 1.5 litres water ● Protective Nutrients Formula ● Skin, Hair, Nails Formula ● Used plant-oil based products	
SATURDAY ☐ Exercise ☐ Eating Plan ☐ Supplement ☐ Skincare	● 2-3 x 5-7 min rebounding ● Walked 10,000 steps ● Had greens & tomato-based dish ● Drank 1.5 litres water ● Protective Nutrients Formula ● Skin, Hair, Nails Formula ● Used plant-oil based products	
SUNDAY ☐ Exercise ☐ Eating Plan ☐ Supplement ☐ Skincare	● 2-3 x 5-7 min rebounding ● Walked 10,000 steps ● Had greens & tomato-based dish ● Drank 1.5 litres water ● Protective Nutrients Formula ● Skin, Hair, Nails Formula ● Used plant-oil based products	

Week Two

INSPIRATION: 'I wouldn't dream of starting the day until I have taken my morning dose of youth elixir – exercise.'
Ginger Rogers, aged 60

Helpful hints: Eat only when you're truly hungry. Don't eat because you're bored, depressed, others want you to, it's time, it's there, or you paid for it. If you eat because you're upset, make a list of alternative actions you can take instead of eating when you're not really hungry.

If you have a pudding, have it after a meal and don't make it the meal or snack. Make sure it doesn't contain hydrogenated fat, limit it to once a week, and remember to savour it, enjoy it, and not feel guilty about having eaten it.

DAY			NOTES
MONDAY			
☐ Exercise	● 1-2 x 10 mins rebounding	● Walked 10,000 steps	
☐ Eating Plan	● Had greens & tomato-based dish	● Drank 1.5 litres water	
☐ Supplement	● Protective Nutrients Formula	● Skin, Hair, Nails Formula	
☐ Skincare	● Used plant-oil based products		
TUESDAY			
☐ Exercise	● 1-2 x 10 mins rebounding	● Walked 10,000 steps	
☐ Eating Plan	● Had greens & tomato-based dish	● Drank 1.5 litres water	
☐ Supplement	● Protective Nutrients Formula	● Skin, Hair, Nails Formula	
☐ Skincare	● Used plant-oil based products		
WEDNESDAY			
☐ Exercise	● 1-2 x 10 mins rebounding	● Walked 10,000 steps	
☐ Eating Plan	● Had greens & tomato-based dish	● Drank 1.5 litres water	
☐ Supplement	● Protective Nutrients Formula	● Skin, Hair, Nails Formula	
☐ Skincare	● Used plant-oil based products		
THURSDAY			
☐ Exercise	● 1-2 x 10 mins rebounding	● Walked 10,000 steps	
☐ Eating Plan	● Had greens & tomato-based dish	● Drank 1.5 litres water	
☐ Supplement	● Protective Nutrients Formula	● Skin, Hair, Nails Formula	
☐ Skincare	● Used plant-oil based products		
FRIDAY			
☐ Exercise	● 1-2 x 10 min rebounding	● Walked 10,000 steps	
☐ Eating Plan	● Had greens & tomato-based dish	● Drank 1.5 litres water	
☐ Supplement	● Protective Nutrients Formula	● Skin, Hair, Nails Formula	
☐ Skincare	● Used plant-oil based products		
SATURDAY			
☐ Exercise	● 1-2 x 10 min rebounding	● Walked 10,000 steps	
☐ Eating Plan	● Had greens & tomato-based dish	● Drank 1.5 litres water	
☐ Supplement	● Protective Nutrients Formula	● Skin, Hair, Nails Formula	
☐ Skincare	● Used plant-oil based products		
SUNDAY			
☐ Exercise	● 1-2 x 10 min rebounding	● Walked 10,000 steps	
☐ Eating Plan	● Had greens & tomato-based dish	● Drank 1.5 litres water	
☐ Supplement	● Protective Nutrients Formula	● Skin, Hair, Nails Formula	
☐ Skincare	● Used plant-oil based products		

Week Three

INSPIRATION:

'You're never too old to become younger.'
Mae West

Helpful hints: Concentrate on finding personal measures of improvement. Are you feeling better, or looking better? Are you receiving positive comments? Remember to stay off the scales because muscle weighs more than fat and you are increasing your muscle mass. If you must, weigh yourself only once a fortnight.

Use a 'trigger' for your rebounding, either every time you hear a news bulletin, or every time a soap is on, get on the rebounder.

DAY			NOTES
MONDAY			
☐ Exercise	● 1-2 x 15 min rebounding	● Walked 10,000 steps	
☐ Eating Plan	● Had greens & tomato-based dish	● Drank 1.5 litres water	
☐ Supplement	● Protective Nutrients Formula	● Skin, Hair, Nails Formula	
☐ Skincare	● Used plant-oil based products		
TUESDAY			
☐ Exercise	● 1-2 x 15 min rebounding	● Walked 10,000 steps	
☐ Eating Plan	● Had greens & tomato-based dish	● Drank 1.5 litres water	
☐ Supplement	● Protective Nutrients Formula	● Skin, Hair, Nails Formula	
☐ Skincare	● Used plant-oil based products		
WEDNESDAY			
☐ Exercise	● 1-2 x 15 min rebounding	● Walked 10,000 steps	
☐ Eating Plan	● Had greens & tomato-based dish	● Drank 1.5 litres water	
☐ Supplement	● Protective Nutrients Formula	● Skin, Hair, Nails Formula	
☐ Skincare	● Used plant-oil based products		
THURSDAY			
☐ Exercise	● 1-2 x 15 min rebounding	● Walked 10,000 steps	
☐ Eating Plan	● Had greens & tomato-based dish	● Drank 1.5 litres water	
☐ Supplement	● Protective Nutrients Formula	● Skin, Hair, Nails Formula	
☐ Skincare	● Used plant-oil based products		
FRIDAY			
☐ Exercise	● 1-2 x 15 min rebounding	● Walked 10,000 steps	
☐ Eating Plan	● Had greens & tomato-based dish	● Drank 1.5 litres water	
☐ Supplement	● Protective Nutrients Formula	● Skin, Hair, Nails Formula	
☐ Skincare	● Used plant-oil based products		
SATURDAY			
☐ Exercise	● 1-2 x 15 min rebounding	● Walked 10,000 steps	
☐ Eating Plan	● Had greens & tomato-based dish	● Drank 1.5 litres water	
☐ Supplement	● Protective Nutrients Formula	● Skin, Hair, Nails Formula	
☐ Skincare	● Used plant-oil based products		
SUNDAY			
☐ Exercise	● 1-2 x 15 min rebounding	● Walked 10,000 steps	
☐ Eating Plan	● Had greens & tomato-based dish	● Drank 1.5 litres water	
☐ Supplement	● Protective Nutrients Formula	● Skin, Hair, Nails Formula	
☐ Skincare	● Used plant-oil based products		

Week Four

INSPIRATION:

'Motivation is what gets you started. Habit is what keeps you going.'
Horace

Helpful hints: When you feel like doing nothing, do a little. Many programmes are abandoned because the 30 minute workout seems like too much and you end up doing nothing. On days like this, change your goal to 15, 10, or even 5 minutes, but just do something. Consistently doing 5 minutes of rebounding is better than doing 20 minutes every so often.

A simple rule for eating a diet high in antioxidant-rich foods effortlessly – give yourself extra portions of vegetables with every meal.

DAY		NOTES
MONDAY		
☐ Exercise	● 1-2 x 20 min rebounding ● Walked 10,000 steps	
☐ Eating Plan	● Had greens & tomato-based dish ● Drank 1.5 litres water	
☐ Supplement	● Protective Nutrients Formula ● Skin, Hair, Nails Formula	
☐ Skincare	● Used plant-oil based products	
TUESDAY		
☐ Exercise	● 1-2 x 20 min rebounding ● Walked 10,000 steps	
☐ Eating Plan	● Had greens & tomato-based dish ● Drank 1.5 litres water	
☐ Supplement	● Protective Nutrients Formula ● Skin, Hair, Nails Formula	
☐ Skincare	● Used plant-oil based products	
WEDNESDAY		
☐ Exercise	● 1-2 x 20 min rebounding ● Walked 10,000 steps	
☐ Eating Plan	● Had greens & tomato-based dish ● Drank 1.5 litres water	
☐ Supplement	● Protective Nutrients Formula ● Skin, Hair, Nails Formula	
☐ Skincare	● Used plant-oil based products	
THURSDAY		
☐ Exercise	● 1-2 x 20 min rebounding ● Walked 10,000 steps	
☐ Eating Plan	● Had greens & tomato-based dish ● Drank 1.5 litres water	
☐ Supplement	● Protective Nutrients Formula ● Skin, Hair, Nails Formula	
☐ Skincare	● Used plant-oil based products	
FRIDAY		
☐ Exercise	● 1-2 x 20 min rebounding ● Walked 10,000 steps	
☐ Eating Plan	● Had greens & tomato-based dish ● Drank 1.5 litres water	
☐ Supplement	● Protective Nutrients Formula ● Skin, Hair, Nails Formula	
☐ Skincare	● Used plant-oil based products	
SATURDAY		
☐ Exercise	● 1-2 x 20 min rebounding ● Walked 10,000 steps	
☐ Eating Plan	● Had greens & tomato-based dish ● Drank 1.5 litres water	
☐ Supplement	● Protective Nutrients Formula ● Skin, Hair, Nails Formula	
☐ Skincare	● Used plant-oil based products	
SUNDAY		
☐ Exercise	● 1-2 x 20 min rebounding ● Walked 10,000 steps	
☐ Eating Plan	● Had greens & tomato-based dish ● Drank 1.5 litres water	
☐ Supplement	● Protective Nutrients Formula ● Skin, Hair, Nails Formula	
☐ Skincare	● Used plant-oil based products	

Week Five

INSPIRATION: 'What lies behind us and what lies before us are small matters compared to what lies within us.'
Ralph Waldo Emerson

Helpful hints: Drink green tea regularly. It's full of antioxidants and can help the body burn fat. If you're getting bored, change your workout. Go for regular walks.

And try to end meals with something savoury. Either have this in place of pudding, or, if it's a special occasion, have the pudding then something savoury because ending a meal with something sweet often makes you crave more sweets.

DAY			NOTES
MONDAY			
☐ Exercise	● 1 x 20 min rebounding	● Walked 10,000 steps	
☐ Eating Plan	● Had greens & tomato-based dish	● Drank 1.5 litres water	
☐ Supplement	● Protective Nutrients Formula	● Skin, Hair, Nails Formula	
☐ Skincare	● Used plant-oil based products		
TUESDAY			
☐ Exercise	● 1 x 20 min rebounding	● Walked 10,000 steps	
☐ Eating Plan	● Had greens & tomato-based dish	● Drank 1.5 litres water	
☐ Supplement	● Protective Nutrients Formula	● Skin, Hair, Nails Formula	
☐ Skincare	● Used plant-oil based products		
WEDNESDAY			
☐ Exercise	● 1 x 20 min rebounding	● Walked 10,000 steps	
☐ Eating Plan	● Had greens & tomato-based dish	● Drank 1.5 litres water	
☐ Supplement	● Protective Nutrients Formula	● Skin, Hair, Nails Formula	
☐ Skincare	● Used plant-oil based products		
THURSDAY			
☐ Exercise	● 1 x 20 min rebounding	● Walked 10,000 steps	
☐ Eating Plan	● Had greens & tomato-based dish	● Drank 1.5 litres water	
☐ Supplement	● Protective Nutrients Formula	● Skin, Hair, Nails Formula	
☐ Skincare	● Used plant-oil based products		
FRIDAY			
☐ Exercise	● 1 x 20 min rebounding	● Walked 10,000 steps	
☐ Eating Plan	● Had greens & tomato-based dish	● Drank 1.5 litres water	
☐ Supplement	● Protective Nutrients Formula	● Skin, Hair, Nails Formula	
☐ Skincare	● Used plant-oil based products		
SATURDAY			
☐ Exercise	● 1 x 20 min rebounding	● Walked 10,000 steps	
☐ Eating Plan	● Had greens & tomato-based dish	● Drank 1.5 litres water	
☐ Supplement	● Protective Nutrients Formula	● Skin, Hair, Nails Formula	
☐ Skincare	● Used plant-oil based products		
SUNDAY			
☐ Exercise	● 1 x 20 min rebounding	● Walked 10,000 steps	
☐ Eating Plan	● Had greens & tomato-based dish	● Drank 1.5 litres water	
☐ Supplement	● Protective Nutrients Formula	● Skin, Hair, Nails Formula	
☐ Skincare	● Used plant-oil based products		

Week Six

INSPIRATION:

'Expecting something for nothing is the most popular form of hope.'
Arnold H. Glasgow

Helpful hints: Whenever you feel tempted to reach for the biscuits or something sweet, brush your teeth. You are less likely to eat something sweet with a fresh, minty mouth.

And have a glass of water at least 30 minutes before every meal, and at least 30 minutes after, that way you've already had nearly all of your water intake for the day without even trying.

DAY		NOTES
MONDAY		
☐ Exercise	● 1 x 20 min rebounding ● Walked 10,000 steps	
☐ Eating Plan	● Had greens & tomato-based dish ● Drank 1.5 litres water	
☐ Supplement	● Protective Nutrients Formula ● Skin, Hair, Nails Formula	
☐ Skincare	● Used plant-oil based products	
TUESDAY		
☐ Exercise	● 1 x 20 min rebounding ● Walked 10,000 steps	
☐ Eating Plan	● Had greens & tomato-based dish ● Drank 1.5 litres water	
☐ Supplement	● Protective Nutrients Formula ● Skin, Hair, Nails Formula	
☐ Skincare	● Used plant-oil based products	
WEDNESDAY		
☐ Exercise	● 1 x 20 min rebounding ● Walked 10,000 steps	
☐ Eating Plan	● Had greens & tomato-based dish ● Drank 1.5 litres water	
☐ Supplement	● Protective Nutrients Formula ● Skin, Hair, Nails Formula	
☐ Skincare	● Used plant-oil based products	
THURSDAY		
☐ Exercise	● 1 x 20 min rebounding ● Walked 10,000 steps	
☐ Eating Plan	● Had greens & tomato-based dish ● Drank 1.5 litres water	
☐ Supplement	● Protective Nutrients Formula ● Skin, Hair, Nails Formula	
☐ Skincare	● Used plant-oil based products	
FRIDAY		
☐ Exercise	● 1 x 20 min rebounding ● Walked 10,000 steps	
☐ Eating Plan	● Had greens & tomato-based dish ● Drank 1.5 litres water	
☐ Supplement	● Protective Nutrients Formula ● Skin, Hair, Nails Formula	
☐ Skincare	● Used plant-oil based products	
SATURDAY		
☐ Exercise	● 1 x 20 min rebounding ● Walked 10,000 steps	
☐ Eating Plan	● Had greens & tomato-based dish ● Drank 1.5 litres water	
☐ Supplement	● Protective Nutrients Formula ● Skin, Hair, Nails Formula	
☐ Skincare	● Used plant-oil based products	
SUNDAY		
☐ Exercise	● 1 x 20 min rebounding ● Walked 10,000 steps	
☐ Eating Plan	● Had greens & tomato-based dish ● Drank 1.5 litres water	
☐ Supplement	● Protective Nutrients Formula ● Skin, Hair, Nails Formula	
☐ Skincare	● Used plant-oil based products	

Week Seven

INSPIRATION:

'The only place you'll find success before work is in the dictionary.'

May B. Smith

Helpful hints: Keep in mind the big picture. There are 168 hours in a week and you will need to rebound for between and 1 and 3 of them during your time on the plan to reap the benefits

DAY		NOTES
MONDAY		
☐ Exercise ● 1 x 25 min rebounding ● Walked 10,000 steps		
☐ Eating Plan ● Had greens & tomato-based dish ● Drank 1.5 litres water		
☐ Supplement ● Protective Nutrients Formula ● Skin, Hair, Nails Formula		
☐ Skincare ● Used plant-oil based products		
TUESDAY		
☐ Exercise ● 1 x 25 min rebounding ● Walked 10,000 steps		
☐ Eating Plan ● Had greens & tomato-based dish ● Drank 1.5 litres water		
☐ Supplement ● Protective Nutrients Formula ● Skin, Hair, Nails Formula		
☐ Skincare ● Used plant-oil based products		
WEDNESDAY		
☐ Exercise ● 1 x 25 min rebounding ● Walked 10,000 steps		
☐ Eating Plan ● Had greens & tomato-based dish ● Drank 1.5 litres water		
☐ Supplement ● Protective Nutrients Formula ● Skin, Hair, Nails Formula		
☐ Skincare ● Used plant-oil based products		
THURSDAY		
☐ Exercise ● 1 x 25 min rebounding ● Walked 10,000 steps		
☐ Eating Plan ● Had greens & tomato-based dish ● Drank 1.5 litres water		
☐ Supplement ● Protective Nutrients Formula ● Skin, Hair, Nails Formula		
☐ Skincare ● Used plant-oil based products		
FRIDAY		
☐ Exercise ● 1 x 25 min rebounding ● Walked 10,000 steps		
☐ Eating Plan ● Had greens & tomato-based dish ● Drank 1.5 litres water		
☐ Supplement ● Protective Nutrients Formula ● Skin, Hair, Nails Formula		
☐ Skincare ● Used plant-oil based products		
SATURDAY		
☐ Exercise ● 1 x 25 min rebounding ● Walked 10,000 steps		
☐ Eating Plan ● Had greens & tomato-based dish ● Drank 1.5 litres water		
☐ Supplement ● Protective Nutrients Formula ● Skin, Hair, Nails Formula		
☐ Skincare ● Used plant-oil based products		
SUNDAY		
☐ Exercise ● 1 x 25 min rebounding ● Walked 10,000 steps		
☐ Eating Plan ● Had greens & tomato-based dish ● Drank 1.5 litres water		
☐ Supplement ● Protective Nutrients Formula ● Skin, Hair, Nails Formula		
☐ Skincare ● Used plant-oil based products		

Week Eight

INSPIRATION: 'The tragedy of life doesn't lie in not reaching your goal. The tragedy lies in having no goal to reach.'
Benjamin E. Mays

Helpful hints: When rebounding, don't answer the phone, or put on the answering machine, put on your favourite up-tempo record, and when you feel like doing nothing, do something. Make it fun. Exercise to music, and let the children have a go.

DAY			NOTES
MONDAY			
☐ Exercise	● 1 x 25 min rebounding	● Walked 10,000 steps	
☐ Eating Plan	● Had greens & tomato-based dish	● Drank 1.5 litres water	
☐ Supplement	● Protective Nutrients Formula	● Skin, Hair, Nails Formula	
☐ Skincare	● Used plant-oil based products		
TUESDAY			
☐ Exercise	● 1 x 25 min rebounding	● Walked 10,000 steps	
☐ Eating Plan	● Had greens & tomato-based dish	● Drank 1.5 litres water	
☐ Supplement	● Protective Nutrients Formula	● Skin, Hair, Nails Formula	
☐ Skincare	● Used plant-oil based products		
WEDNESDAY			
☐ Exercise	● 1 x 25 min rebounding	● Walked 10,000 steps	
☐ Eating Plan	● Had greens & tomato-based dish	● Drank 1.5 litres water	
☐ Supplement	● Protective Nutrients Formula	● Skin, Hair, Nails Formula	
☐ Skincare	● Used plant-oil based products		
THURSDAY			
☐ Exercise	● 1 x 25 min rebounding	● Walked 10,000 steps	
☐ Eating Plan	● Had greens & tomato-based dish	● Drank 1.5 litres water	
☐ Supplement	● Protective Nutrients Formula	● Skin, Hair, Nails Formula	
☐ Skincare	● Used plant-oil based products		
FRIDAY			
☐ Exercise	● 1 x 25 min rebounding	● Walked 10,000 steps	
☐ Eating Plan	● Had greens & tomato-based dish	● Drank 1.5 litres water	
☐ Supplement	● Protective Nutrients Formula	● Skin, Hair, Nails Formula	
☐ Skincare	● Used plant-oil based products		
SATURDAY			
☐ Exercise	● 1 x 25 min rebounding	● Walked 10,000 steps	
☐ Eating Plan	● Had greens & tomato-based dish	● Drank 1.5 litres water	
☐ Supplement	● Protective Nutrients Formula	● Skin, Hair, Nails Formula	
☐ Skincare	● Used plant-oil based products		
SUNDAY			
☐ Exercise	● 1 x 25 min rebounding	● Walked 10,000 steps	
☐ Eating Plan	● Had greens & tomato-based dish	● Drank 1.5 litres water	
☐ Supplement	● Protective Nutrients Formula	● Skin, Hair, Nails Formula	
☐ Skincare	● Used plant-oil based products		

Week Nine

INSPIRATION:

'If you want to be a picture of health, you'd better have a happy frame of min.' Unknown

Helpful hints: Get in a comfortable position. Relax, take a few deep breaths and close your eyes. Picture each cell in your body strengthening as the body feels the effects of consistently exercising on your rebounder. Picture each cell taking just what it needs and all the excess fat, fluid and toxins dropping off. See your connective tissue strengthening as your body becomes strong, vibrant, detoxified, toned, and youthful.

DAY			NOTES
MONDAY			
☐ Exercise	● 1 x 25 min rebounding	● Walked 10,000 steps	
☐ Eating Plan	● Had greens & tomato-based dish	● Drank 1.5 litres water	
☐ Supplement	● Protective Nutrients Formula	● Skin, Hair, Nails Formula	
☐ Skincare	● Used plant-oil based products		
TUESDAY			
☐ Exercise	● 1 x 25 min rebounding	● Walked 10,000 steps	
☐ Eating Plan	● Had greens & tomato-based dish	● Drank 1.5 litres water	
☐ Supplement	● Protective Nutrients Formula	● Skin, Hair, Nails Formula	
☐ Skincare	● Used plant-oil based products		
WEDNESDAY			
☐ Exercise	● 1 x 25 min rebounding	● Walked 10,000 steps	
☐ Eating Plan	● Had greens & tomato-based dish	● Drank 1.5 litres water	
☐ Supplement	● Protective Nutrients Formula	● Skin, Hair, Nails Formula	
☐ Skincare	● Used plant-oil based products		
THURSDAY			
☐ Exercise	● 1 x 25 min rebounding	● Walked 10,000 steps	
☐ Eating Plan	● Had greens & tomato-based dish	● Drank 1.5 litres water	
☐ Supplement	● Protective Nutrients Formula	● Skin, Hair, Nails Formula	
☐ Skincare	● Used plant-oil based products		
FRIDAY			
☐ Exercise	● 1 x 25 min rebounding	● Walked 10,000 steps	
☐ Eating Plan	● Had greens & tomato-based dish	● Drank 1.5 litres water	
☐ Supplement	● Protective Nutrients Formula	● Skin, Hair, Nails Formula	
☐ Skincare	● Used plant-oil based products		
SATURDAY			
☐ Exercise	● 1 x 25 min rebounding	● Walked 10,000 steps	
☐ Eating Plan	● Had greens & tomato-based dish	● Drank 1.5 litres water	
☐ Supplement	● Protective Nutrients Formula	● Skin, Hair, Nails Formula	
☐ Skincare	● Used plant-oil based products		
SUNDAY			
☐ Exercise	● 1 x 25 min rebounding	● Walked 10,000 steps	
☐ Eating Plan	● Had greens & tomato-based dish	● Drank 1.5 litres water	
☐ Supplement	● Protective Nutrients Formula	● Skin, Hair, Nails Formula	
☐ Skincare	● Used plant-oil based products		

Week Ten

INSPIRATION:

'Without knowledge we perish.'
The Bible

Helpful hints: Educate yourself as much as possible. We are all intuitively guided to do what is right for us, and you will soon unlearn a lot of bad habits.

DAY		NOTES
MONDAY		
☐ Exercise	● 1 x 30 min rebounding ● Walked 10,000 steps	
☐ Eating Plan	● Had greens & tomato-based dish ● Drank 1.5 litres water	
☐ Supplement	● Protective Nutrients Formula ● Skin, Hair, Nails Formula	
☐ Skincare	● Used plant-oil based products	
TUESDAY		
☐ Exercise	● 1 x 30 min rebounding ● Walked 10,000 steps	
☐ Eating Plan	● Had greens & tomato-based dish ● Drank 1.5 litres water	
☐ Supplement	● Protective Nutrients Formula ● Skin, Hair, Nails Formula	
☐ Skincare	● Used plant-oil based products	
WEDNESDAY		
☐ Exercise	● 1 x 30 min rebounding ● Walked 10,000 steps	
☐ Eating Plan	● Had greens & tomato-based dish ● Drank 1.5 litres water	
☐ Supplement	● Protective Nutrients Formula ● Skin, Hair, Nails Formula	
☐ Skincare	● Used plant-oil based products	
THURSDAY		
☐ Exercise	● 1 x 30 min rebounding ● Walked 10,000 steps	
☐ Eating Plan	● Had greens & tomato-based dish ● Drank 1.5 litres water	
☐ Supplement	● Protective Nutrients Formula ● Skin, Hair, Nails Formula	
☐ Skincare	● Used plant-oil based products	
FRIDAY		
☐ Exercise	● 1 x 30 min rebounding ● Walked 10,000 steps	
☐ Eating Plan	● Had greens & tomato-based dish ● Drank 1.5 litres water	
☐ Supplement	● Protective Nutrients Formula ● Skin, Hair, Nails Formula	
☐ Skincare	● Used plant-oil based products	
SATURDAY		
☐ Exercise	● 1 x 30 min rebounding ● Walked 10,000 steps	
☐ Eating Plan	● Had greens & tomato-based dish ● Drank 1.5 litres water	
☐ Supplement	● Protective Nutrients Formula ● Skin, Hair, Nails Formula	
☐ Skincare	● Used plant-oil based products	
SUNDAY		
☐ Exercise	● 1 x 30 min rebounding ● Walked 10,000 steps	
☐ Eating Plan	● Had greens & tomato-based dish ● Drank 1.5 litres water	
☐ Supplement	● Protective Nutrients Formula ● Skin, Hair, Nails Formula	
☐ Skincare	● Used plant-oil based products	

Week Eleven

INSPIRATION: 'The body is a sacred garment. It is your first and last garment, it is what you enter life in and what you depart life with, and it should be treated with honour.' Martha Graham

Helpful hints: Read labels of everything that you buy for consumption and a good general rule is: if it contains anything hydrogenated or partially hydrogenated, or if the list of ingredients goes on for over four lines (meaning that it's probably full of artificial sweeteners, preservatives, colourings and other chemicals), don't buy it.

DAY		NOTES
MONDAY		
☐ **Exercise** ● 1 x 30 min rebounding ● Walked 10,000 steps		
☐ **Eating Plan** ● Had greens & tomato-based dish ● Drank 1.5 litres water		
☐ **Supplement** ● Protective Nutrients Formula ● Skin, Hair, Nails Formula		
☐ **Skincare** ● Used plant-oil based products		
TUESDAY		
☐ **Exercise** ● 1 x 30 min rebounding ● Walked 10,000 steps		
☐ **Eating Plan** ● Had greens & tomato-based dish ● Drank 1.5 litres water		
☐ **Supplement** ● Protective Nutrients Formula ● Skin, Hair, Nails Formula		
☐ **Skincare** ● Used plant-oil based products		
WEDNESDAY		
☐ **Exercise** ● 1 x 30 min rebounding ● Walked 10,000 steps		
☐ **Eating Plan** ● Had greens & tomato-based dish ● Drank 1.5 litres water		
☐ **Supplement** ● Protective Nutrients Formula ● Skin, Hair, Nails Formula		
☐ **Skincare** ● Used plant-oil based products		
THURSDAY		
☐ **Exercise** ● 1 x 30 min rebounding ● Walked 10,000 steps		
☐ **Eating Plan** ● Had greens & tomato-based dish ● Drank 1.5 litres water		
☐ **Supplement** ● Protective Nutrients Formula ● Skin, Hair, Nails Formula		
☐ **Skincare** ● Used plant-oil based products		
FRIDAY		
☐ **Exercise** ● 1 x 30 min rebounding ● Walked 10,000 steps		
☐ **Eating Plan** ● Had greens & tomato-based dish ● Drank 1.5 litres water		
☐ **Supplement** ● Protective Nutrients Formula ● Skin, Hair, Nails Formula		
☐ **Skincare** ● Used plant-oil based products		
SATURDAY		
☐ **Exercise** ● 1 x 30 min rebounding ● Walked 10,000 steps		
☐ **Eating Plan** ● Had greens & tomato-based dish ● Drank 1.5 litres water		
☐ **Supplement** ● Protective Nutrients Formula ● Skin, Hair, Nails Formula		
☐ **Skincare** ● Used plant-oil based products		
SUNDAY		
☐ **Exercise** ● 1 x 30 min rebounding ● Walked 10,000 steps		
☐ **Eating Plan** ● Had greens & tomato-based dish ● Drank 1.5 litres water		
☐ **Supplement** ● Protective Nutrients Formula ● Skin, Hair, Nails Formula		
☐ **Skincare** ● Used plant-oil based products		

Week Twelve

INSPIRATION:

'Well done is better than well said.'
Benjamin Franklin

Helpful hints: Don't overeat. Buy smaller dinner plates – you'll soon get used to eating smaller portions. And always stop when you're full, despite being trained as a child to finish your plate.

DAY		NOTES
MONDAY		
☐ Exercise	● 1 x 30 min rebounding ● Walked 10,000 steps	
☐ Eating Plan	● Had greens & tomato-based dish ● Drank 1.5 litres water	
☐ Supplement	● Protective Nutrients Formula ● Skin, Hair, Nails Formula	
☐ Skincare	● Used plant-oil based products	
TUESDAY		
☐ Exercise	● 1 x 30 min rebounding ● Walked 10,000 steps	
☐ Eating Plan	● Had greens & tomato-based dish ● Drank 1.5 litres water	
☐ Supplement	● Protective Nutrients Formula ● Skin, Hair, Nails Formula	
☐ Skincare	● Used plant-oil based products	
WEDNESDAY		
☐ Exercise	● 1 x 30 min rebounding ● Walked 10,000 steps	
☐ Eating Plan	● Had greens & tomato-based dish ● Drank 1.5 litres water	
☐ Supplement	● Protective Nutrients Formula ● Skin, Hair, Nails Formula	
☐ Skincare	● Used plant-oil based products	
THURSDAY		
☐ Exercise	● 1 x 30 min rebounding ● Walked 10,000 steps	
☐ Eating Plan	● Had greens & tomato-based dish ● Drank 1.5 litres water	
☐ Supplement	● Protective Nutrients Formula ● Skin, Hair, Nails Formula	
☐ Skincare	● Used plant-oil based products	
FRIDAY		
☐ Exercise	● 1 x 30 min rebounding ● Walked 10,000 steps	
☐ Eating Plan	● Had greens & tomato-based dish ● Drank 1.5 litres water	
☐ Supplement	● Protective Nutrients Formula ● Skin, Hair, Nails Formula	
☐ Skincare	● Used plant-oil based products	
SATURDAY		
☐ Exercise	● 1 x 30 min rebounding ● Walked 10,000 steps	
☐ Eating Plan	● Had greens & tomato-based dish ● Drank 1.5 litres water	
☐ Supplement	● Protective Nutrients Formula ● Skin, Hair, Nails Formula	
☐ Skincare	● Used plant-oil based products	
SUNDAY		
☐ Exercise	● 1 x 30 min rebounding ● Walked 10,000 steps	
☐ Eating Plan	● Had greens & tomato-based dish ● Drank 1.5 litres water	
☐ Supplement	● Protective Nutrients Formula ● Skin, Hair, Nails Formula	
☐ Skincare	● Used plant-oil based products	

Resources

All resources mentioned in the Programme can be foundon the website www.nonipsnotucks.com and many can be purchased at discounted prices.

Trimilin Rebounders and support bars
Available from www.nonipsnotucks.com

No Nips No Tucks Anti-ageing Protective Nutrients
No Nips No Tucks Skin, Hair and Nails Formula
Available from www.nonipsnotucks.com

Oleicia Skin and haircare products
Available from www.nonipsnotucks.com

Other skincare recommendations:
Trilogy 100% Rosehip Oil
Weleda Wild Rose Intensive Facial Oil
Jurlique Day Care Facial Oil
Organic Pharmacy Skin Rescue Oil
Neals Yard Jasmine Skin Nourishing Oil
Aveda Balancing Infusion (for dry skin)
Beauty Without Cruelty Vitamin C Vitality Serum
Jasons Natural Hyper C Serum Anti-aging Therapy
SKIN.NY Radical Restructure Complex (clinically proven to reduce wrinkles)
Lavera Lifting Serum Hydro Gel
Dermalogica - Skin Soothing Cream
Jurlique Wrinkle Skin Softener Beauty cream
Green People Fruitful Nights / Vitamin Fix
Elemis Pro Collagen Quartz Lift Serum
Korres Olive and Rye Night Cream
Living Nature Firming Flax Cream

Symbiotropin – for more information see www.nonipsnotucks.com

Ho Shou Wu – Available from Chinese herbalists
Fleeceflower available from www.nonipsnotucks.com

Oxygen Based Colon Cleanse Products – for more information see www.nonipsnotucks.com

Water Ionizers - www.thewaterioniser.co.uk

MBTs – see www.swissmasai.co.uk for retailers

Omron Pedometers (I recommend the Walking Style II) from Omron Healthcare Ltd,
Tel: 01908 258285

IJoyRide see link on www.nonipsnotucks.com

Anti-oxidant testing for more information see www.nonipsnotucks.com

Teeth whitening – London Cosmetic Dentistry www.londoncosmeticdentistry.co.uk

References

Why and how we age

1. Rudman D, Feller AG, Cohn L, Shetty KR, Rudman IW, Draper MW (1991) Effects of human growth hormone on body composition in elderly men. Horm Res 36 (Suppl 1):73–81
2. Cohn L, Feller AG, Draper MW, Rudman IW, Rudman D (1993) Carpal tunnel syndrome and gynaecomastia during growth hormone treatment of elderly men with low circulating IGF-I concentrations. Clin Endocrinol (Oxf) 39(4):417–25
3. Jamieson J, Dorman LE (1997) The role of somatotroph-specific peptides and IGF-1 intermediate as an alternative to HGH injections. AmColl Adv Med Oct
4. Diamond P et al. (1996) Metabolic effects of 12 month percutaneous DHEA replacement therapy in post-menopausal women. J Endocrinol 150:43–50
5. Khorram O, Vu L, Yen S (1997) Activation of immune function by DHEA in age-advanced men. J Gerontol 52A(1):M1–M7
6. Wolkowitz O et al. (1997) DHEA treatment of depression. Biol Psychiat 41:311–18
7. Sreekumaran Nair K, Rizza R, O'Brien P et al. (2006) DHEA in elderly women and DHEA or testosterone in elderly men. New Engl J Med 355:1647–59

The anti-ageing eating plan

1. Sander CS et al. (2002) Photoageing is associated with protein oxidation in human skin in vivo. J Invest Dermatol 118:618–25
2. Watkins BA, Seifert MF (1996) Food lipids and bone health. In: Food Lipids and Health (eds RE McDonald, DB Min). New York NY: Marcel Dekker, Inc, p
3. Nanji AA et al. (1995) Gastroenterology 109(2):547–54; Cha YS, Sachan DS (1994) J Am Coll Nutr 13(4):338–43
4. Kabara JJ (1978) The Pharmacological Effects of Lipids. Champaign IL: The American Oil Chemists Society, pp. 1–14
4. Cohen LA et al. (1986) J Natl Cancer Inst 77:43
5. Pinckney E, Pinckney C (1973) The Cholesterol Controversy. Los Angeles: Sherbourne Press, pp. 127–131, Research indicating the correlation of polyunsaturates with learning problems. In: Harmon D et al. (1976) J Am Geriatrics Soc 24(1):292–8, Meerson Z et al. (1983) Bull Exp Biol Med 96(9):7071, Valero et al. (1990) Regarding weight gain, levels of linoleic acid in adipose tissues reflect the amount of linoleic acid in the diet. Ann Nutr Metabol 34(6):323–7, Felton CV et al. (1994) Lancet 344:1195–6
6. Okuyama H et al. (1997) Prog Lipid Res 35(4):409–57

The exercise plan that keeps you youthful

1. Seguin R, Nelson ME (2003) The benefits of strength training for older adults. Am Prev Med 25(Suppl 2):S14–9
2. Bhattacharya E, McCutcheon E, Shvariz E, Greenleaf J (1980) J Appl Physiol 49(5):881–7

Anti-ageing haircare

1. Military Academy of Medical Scientific Research in Toxicology (1994) Immunophar macology of Chinese Herbal Medicine. Beijing: People's Army Medical Corp., pp. 1053–70
2. (1993) Advances in the research on the pharmacology of He Shou Wu. Chinese

Materia Medica 16(2):34–7

3. (1994) Medicine of American Digest. Link Publications, Kenneth Baker Edward, Research and Findings 5:234–42

Anti-ageing nutrients

1. Bast A, Haenen GR. (1988) Interplay between lipoic acid and glutathione in the protection against microsomal lipid peroxidation. Biochim Biophys Acta 16;963(3):558–61

2. Packer L, Witt EH, Tritschler HJ (1995) Alpha-lipoic acid as a biological antioxidant. Free Radic Biol Med 19(2):227–50

3. Packer L, Tritschler HJ, Wessel K (1997) Neuroprotection by the metabolic antioxidant alpha-lipoic acid. Free Radic Biol Med 22(1–2):359–78

4. Packer L, Kraemer K, Rimbach G (2001) Molecular aspects of lipoic acid in the prevention of diabetes complications. Nutrition 17(10):888–95

5. Liu J, Killilea DW, Ames BN (2002) Age-associated mitochondrial oxidative decay: improvement of carnitine acetyltransferase substrate-binding affinity and activity in brain by feeding old rats acetyl-L-carnitine and/or R-alpha-lipoic acid. Proc Natl Acad Sci USA 19;99(4):1876–81

6. Bruno G, Scaccianoce S, Bonamini M et al. (1995) Acetyl-L-carnitine in Alzheimer disease: a short-term study on CSF neurotransmitters and neuropeptides. Alzheimer Dis Assoc Disord 9(3):128–31

7. Dhitavat S, Ortiz D, Shea TB, Rivera ER (2002) Acetyl-L-carnitine protects against amyloid-beta neurotoxicity: roles of oxidative buffering and ATP levels. Neurochem Res 27(6):501–5

8. Crane FL (2001) Biochemical functions of coenzyme Q10. J Am Coll Nutr 20(6):591–8

9. Hofman-Bang C, Rehnqvist N et al. (1995) Coenzyme Q10 as an adjunctive in the treatment of chronic congestive heart failure. The Q10 Study Group. J Card Fail 1(2):101–7

10. Morisco C, Trimarco B et al. (1993) Effect of Coenzyme Q10 therapy in patients with congestive heart failure: a long-term multicenter randomized study. Clin Invest 71(Suppl. 8):S134–6

11. Singh RB, Niaz MA (1999) Serum concentration of lipoprotein(a) decreases on treatment with hydrosoluble Coenzyme Q10 in patients with coronary artery disease: discovery of a new role. Int J Cardiol 68(1):23–9

12. Singh RB, Niaz MA et al. (1999) Effect of hydrosoluble Coenzyme Q10 on blood pressures and insulin resistance in hypertensive patients with coronary artery disease. J Hum Hypertens 13(3):203–8

13. Langsjoen H, Langsjoen P et al. (1994) Usefulness of Coenzyme Q10 in clinical cardiology: a long-term study. Mol Aspects Med 15(Suppl.):s165–75

14. Davini A, Cellerini F et al. (1992) Coenzyme Q10: contractile dysfunction of the myocardial cell and metabolic therapy. Minerva Cardioangiol 40(11):449–53

15. Mortensen SA, Leth A et al. (1997) Dose related decrease of serum CoQ10 during treatment with HMG-CoA reductase inhibitors. Mol Aspect Med 1(Suppl.):137–44

16. Bargossi AM, Grossi G et al. (1994) Exogenous CoQ10 supplementation prevents plasma ubiquinone reduction induced by the HMG CoA reductase inhibitors. Mol Aspect Med 15(Suppl.):187–93

17. Rosenfeldt FL, Pepe S et al. (1999) Coenzyme Q10 improves the tolerance of the senescent myocardium to aerobic and ischemic stress: studies in rats and in human atrial tissue. Biofactors 9(2–4):291–9

18. Kalen A, Appelkvist EL et al. (1989) Age-related changes in the lipid compositions of rat and human tissues. Lipids 24(7):579–84

19. Hoppe U, Bergemann J et al. (1999) Coenzyme Q10, a cutaneous antioxidant and energizer. Biofactors 9(2–4):371–8 (Review)

20. Langsjoen PH, Langsjoen AM (1999) Overview of the use of CoQ10 in cardiovascular disease. Biofactors 9(2–4):273–84

21. Hertog M, Feskens EJ, Hollman PC, Katan MB, Kromhout D (1993) Dietary antioxidant flavonoids and risk of coronary heart disease: the Zutphen Elderly Study. Lancet 23;342(8878):1007–11

22. Unno K, Takabayashi F, Kishido T, Oku N (2004) Suppressive effect of green tea catechins on morphologic and functional regression of the brain in aged mice with accelerated senescence (SAMP10). Exp Gerontol 39(7):1027–34

23. Tsuneki H, Ishizuka M, Terasawa M, Wu JB, Sasaoka T, Kimura I (2004) Effect of green tea on blood glucose levels and serum proteomic patterns in diabetic (db/db) mice and on glucose metabolism in healthy humans. BMC Pharmacol 4(1):18

24. Masquelier J (1991) Historical note on OPC. France: Martillac

25. Bagchi D et al. (1998) Protective effects of grape seed proanthocyanidins and selected antioxidants against TPA-induced hepatic and brain lipid peroxidation and DNA fragmentation, and peritoneal macrophage activation in mice. Gen Pharmacol 30(5):771–6

26. Fremont L et al. (1999) Antioxidant activity of resveratrol and alcohol-free wine polyphenols related to LDL oxidation and polyunsaturated fatty acids. Life Sci 64(26):2511–21

27. Ye X, Krohn RL (1999) The cytotoxic effects of a novel IH636 grape seed proanthocyanidin extract on cultured human cancer cells. Mol Cell Biochem 196(1–2):99–108

28. Meunier MT, Villie F (1994) The interaction of Cupressus sempervirens L. proanthocyanidolic oligomers with elastase and elastins. J Pharm Belg 49(6):453–61

29. Carlisle EM (1988) Silicon as a trace nutrient. Sci Total Environ 73:95–106

30. (1995) Silica 57(12): 30

31. Morganti P et al. (1983) Gelatin-cystine keratogenesis and structure of the hair. Boll Soc Ital Biol Sper 59(1):20–5 presume you meant 20–5.

32. Balz F (1999) Antioxidant vitamins and heart disease. Presented at the 60th Annual Biology Colloquium, Oregon State University, Corvallis, Oregon, February 25

33. Wilkinson IB, Megson IL, MacCallum H et al. (1999) Oral vitamin C reduces arterial stiffness and platelet aggregation in humans. J Cardiovasc Pharmacol 34:690–3

34. Levine M, Conry-Cantilena C, Wang Y et al. (1996) Vitamin C pharmacokinetics in healthy volunteers: evidence for a recommended dietary allowance. Proc Natl Acad Sci 93:3704–9

35. Murad H et al. (2001) The effect of an oral supplement containing glucosamine, amino acids, minerals, and antioxidants on cutaneous aging: a preliminary study. J Dermatolog Treat 12(1):47–51

36. Boman G, Backer U, Larsson S, Melander B, Wahlander L (1983) Oral acetylcysteine reduces exacerbation rate in chronic bronchitis: a report of a trial organized by the Swedish Society for Pulmonary Diseases. Eur J Respir Dis 64(6):405–15

37. Zs-Nagy I (2002) Pharmacological interventions against aging through the cell plasma membrane: a review of the experimental results obtained in animals and humans. Ann NY Acad Sci 959:308–20

38. Jamieson J, Dorman LE (1997) The role of somatotroph-specific peptides and IGF-1 intermediate as an alternative to HGH injections. Am Coll Adv Med

Other lifestyle factors that affect ageing

1. Epel ES et al. (2004) Accelerated telomere shortening in response to life stress. Proc Nat Acad Sci 101(49):17312–15

Index

Yinka Thomas MSc RNutr.,

Yinka is a holistic nutritionist specialising in anti-ageing and devises comprehensive individual lifestyle modification Programmes for health, fitness, weight-loss, and anti-ageing.

Yinka has a Master of Science degree in Health, Nutrition and Physical Activity from St Mary's University College Surrey, with a research study in anti-ageing science. Her research following on from that into non-invasive methods of preventing and reversing ageing has led to the No Nips No Tucks™ programme.

Yinka has been a consultant for companies such as Mothercare PLC, Savant Health Ltd, and NaturaLife Ltd for whom she has developed and formulated weight-loss and anti-ageing supplements. She has also worked in Public Health for local authorities in London.

Yinka was health, nutrition and wellness adviser on Vitality Television, and has also appeared on the Baby Channel. She's also written *Have a Baby and Look Better than Ever,* a holistic guide to health and wellness during and after pregnancy, and *The XCell Plan* - a holistic guide to eliminating cellulite naturally.

Yinka is registered with the Nutrition Society, and has sat on the Nutrition Society's Fitness to Practice panel.